T

Hidden

Diagnosis

What Doctors Are Missing and
Why You Should Know

The

Hidden

Diagnosis

What Doctors Are Missing and
Why You Should Know

By Dr. Chris Cormier, D.C.

First Edition
10 9 8 7 6 5 4 3 2

Book Cover design by Cathi Stevenson
www.bookcoverexpress.com

Book Edited by Alexis Orgera
email: alexisorgera@mac.com
&
Heather Marsh
www.classicediting.com

Interior Design by Rudy Milanovich and Keith Leon

The Hidden Diagnosis (soft cover):   978-0-9851333-0-6
The Hidden Diagnosis (ebook):   978-0-9851333-1-3
The Hidden Diagnosis (audio book):   978-0-9851333-2-0

Dr. Chris Cormier
Lafayette, Louisiana
www.TheNerveHealthInstitute.com

This book is dedicated to a very special person whose unconditional love and unwavering support has allowed me to become the man I am. Words cannot express my infinite gratitude. I love you.

Dr. Chris Cormier

"What I like about Dr. Cormier is his willingness to always use cutting edge technology. He is also always striving to improve his practice. He has helped me tremendously. I was barely able to walk and after only one adjustment I was almost healed."
- Phillip Reed

"Dr. Cormier combines knowledge with a desire to help each patient achieve the best quality of life possible. After living with back pain for over 50 years, he helps me stay strong and pain free. I take Superfruits GT and love the little pick up it gives me each morning. I also love his staff. They are always kind and helpful."
- Melva Gray

"The things I like most about Dr. Cormier's treatment are the tools he uses for alignment! There are no surprise movements and hardly any discomfort. Dr. Cormier is able to locate troubled areas immediately and treat with very minimal appointments as compared to 20 – 30 appointments with other chiropractors used in the past. He has helped me tremendously! I no longer have pain in my neck or arms and am able to sleep at night. Dr. Cormier and his staff are awesome! I know that if and when I get any discomfort, I can call Dr. Cormier's office and be seen soon and treated successfully!"
- Janet Ledet

"Dr. Cormier takes the time to talk to me about my pain, what causes it and how he can help me overcome the pain that I might be doing something wrong that causes this pain to be chronic. The methods he uses are very good and simple, which helps me get over whatever pain I might have. He has helped me very, very much. Thank you very much, Dr. Cormier."
- Pat Andrus

"My level of energy and endurance during exercise and afterwards has increased remarkably since undergoing nerve rehabilitation with Dr. Cormier. He has enabled me to maintain

a quality of life that I didn't think I could have as I grew older. Thank you, Dr. Cormier!"
- Phyllis LeBlanc

"Dr. Cormier is very aggressive and passionate about his work. He builds a truly honest and trusting relationship with his patients. His support people are awesome and they get the job done quickly. After two bouts with Parsonage Turner Syndrome, he has improved my upper body strength by 80 percent. I am 59 years old and continue to lead a very active life."
- Al Broussard

"Dr. Cormier uses a natural method of therapy that is absolutely amazing. Before allowing Dr. Cormier to treat me I was averaging six to nine over-the-counter pain medications per day. The medications would ease the pain, but never stop the pain. After a short time of therapy with Dr. Cormier, I am no longer taking any pain medication and 90 percent of the time, I have no pain. My quality of life has improved 110 percent! I can't thank Dr. Cormier enough for treating me. I will be a patient for life."
- Lisa Leon

"Dr. Cormier listens to patients and using his knowledge, ability to research online, articles in magazines, and talks, picks the best approach for an individual patient. Dr. Chris helped me with a back problem using special techniques because of an abdominal aneurism."
- Ralph Domingue

"When I was diagnosed with a pinched nerve in my lower back, I tried everything, including multiple cortisone injections. Luckily, a friend told me about Dr. Cormier and his new techniques of easing back pain. By the end of the second week of treatment, I felt like a new person. I stand erect and walk with no pain; I do things I hadn't been able to do in over a year! I feel he really cares about my overall general health and quality

of life. Also, I've cleansed my body of all synthetic vitamins and impurities and whole-heartedly subscribe to his specially designed Superfruits GT drink. For a 60 year-old woman, I feel 30 thanks to Dr. Cormier!"
- Madge Katsoulis

"Dr. Cormier gets very involved when he is seeing you. I like that he always has a lot of new ideas and techniques to help you. He is very informative and which makes you feel that he really does care about you as a patient. He has helped me out a lot. With the type of work I do I have problems here and there and he always knows what to do to get rid of the problem areas."
- Richlyn Langley

"Dr. Cormier is very serious about his profession. He works on the areas that are hurting, and he knows what he is doing. Dr. Cormier took me on short notice, and he knew what to do to get me back to work. In just three treatments I was able to go back to work with no pain. Before, I was hurting so much that I couldn't hold up my arm. I would recommend him to anybody."
- Glenn Romero

"Dr. Cormier is more than willing to help you with your problems. He is very thorough and understanding. The staff there is awesome. You feel comfortable being there. I am doing much better and feel good. I highly recommend Dr. Cormier and his workers to anyone with pain."
- Fay Lebouef

"I have used traditional medicine in the past and although it helped, it took six to nine months with painful physical therapy. With Dr. Cormier and his staff (and great equipment) I have gotten marked relief within two months. Although I still have room for improvement, two months to feel relief is great compared to six to nine months!"
- Michelle Leger

"Dr. Cormier actually listens to his patients and is very clear with his explanations of what is going on. He cares like you're family. His treatment has helped me so much. I had not realized how much pain I was putting up with until it was gone. I recommend Dr. Cormier to all my family and friends."
- Betty Hebert

"I like Dr. Cormier's positive thinking and honesty. He is also always looking for a better way of helping his patients. He has helped me to live a better lifestyle at my age."
- J.B. Vondenstein

"What I like most about Dr. Cormier is his attention to my personal care and his ability to expand on his expertise through research, study and continuing education. After 15 years of chronic pain and having visited with a multitude of physicians, therapists, and many consultations, I now know what to do when I have a problem or am in need of maintenance…call Dr. Chris!!!"
- Ken Cedotal

"Dr. Cormier is so exciting and progressive in his treatments. He loves what he does and it shows. When I am with him for an appointment, I know I must be his only patient for the day! Dr. Cormier rocks! In short, he gave me back my life."
- Ann Henry

"I like his treatment methodology: natural, clean supplements— NO DRUGS—yeah! He has helped me tremendously. I have zero pain at this moment in time."
- Patty Leger

"Dr. Chris Cormier has really helped me out so much. He is very kind and compassionate about his work. He is also very persistent and will get to the bottom of the problem so his patient can get back to a normal life. When I met Dr. Cormier I told him about my situation. He did all he could do to help me. There

was one thing he told me over and over again when I met with him that really helped me solve my problem and that was to stay away from aspartame. For months I didn't listen to him and, when I finally got off everything that had aspartame, my whole body felt so much better. Thank you, Dr. Cormier. Once I got off aspartame, my body didn't hurt and I didn't have to see Dr. Cormier as much."
- Peggy Vallot

"David and I were impressed with Dr. Cormier's enthusiasm for his profession and his sincerity in helping us resolve health issues and working with us to achieve better quality of health. Our results have been very positive."
- Roberta and David Degeyter

"Dr. Cormier is a real people person. He is one of the most sincere doctors that I have met. He knows how to listen and has a knack for getting to the real root cause of your medical issues. In December of 2008, I started experiencing excruciating pain in the left side of my face and cranium which was later linked to shingles under the skin of my face. This affected the trigeminal nerves and caused great pain. He treated me using Quantum Neurology®, a new method of pain treatment. I had numerous sessions with him at his office which helped manage the pain to a tolerable level. He also treated me at his home on Christmas Eve and Christmas Day. For this man to allow me in his home, especially during these times, I can't express my appreciation enough to Dr. Cormier for helping me through that ordeal."
- Joe Powell

Table of Contents

Dr. Chris Cormier

Acknowledgments

Thanks so much to all.

Words cannot express my sincere gratitude to my amazing wife, Missy, for always being there for me throughout this incredible journey. Without her intuition, support, and constructive criticism, the concepts presented in this book may have never come to fruition.

I also would like to thank thousands of my patients for their unwavering support and for trusting in me to give them the highest level of care possible.

Additionally, I would like to thank my amazing office staff for their support and tireless efforts to help our patients enjoy a higher quality of life.

I would also like to thank Dr. George Gonzalez, founder of Quantum Neurology®, for letting me be a pioneer in the development of this revolutionary nerve rehabilitation technique.

My sincere gratitude also goes to Dr. Edward Chauvin, fellow Quantum Neurologist in Abbeville, Louisiana, for introducing me to Quantum Neurology®, as well as Dr. James Sheen, fellow Quantum Neurologist in Kiarney, Nebraska, for profoundly expanding my knowledge in too many areas to mention.

Thank you to all the leaders and staff at Nature's Liquids for their unwavering support and for allowing me to invent products that people need so desperately.

I would like to thank Alexis Orgera and her incredible writing talents in helping to get everything out of my brain and into this book in a fashion that allows people everywhere to understand the power of the human body through the lens of the nervous system.

Finally, I would like to express sincere gratitude to all the other experts involved in getting this book to you: Keith Leon, Heather Marsh, Glen Clark, Will Bailey, Nicole Hackmann, Amy Jones, Cathi Stevenson, Nate Hackmann, and Rudy Milanovich.

Dr. Chris Cormier

Preface: *clear your bookshelves!*

The idea for this book was born on a family vacation. My family and I recently went to the beach for a week, and our babysitter, Ashley, came along to give my wife and I some much needed alone time. Ashley was not a patient of mine before this trip, but that quickly changed. While in the hotel one day, Ashley developed a terrible headache that rest and darkness wouldn't alleviate. She came to us and asked if we had any over-the-counter painkillers. I don't believe in masking problems, which is exactly what painkillers do. So, instead, with her permission, I neurologically deciphered the reason Ashley's head was hurting and got her back on track. The headache was an alarm going off in her body telling her that there was something wrong with her wiring, some deficiency in the brain that needed fixing. She didn't have a headache because she was low on her painkiller quotient for the month. She wasn't experiencing a deficiency in Advil, Tylenol, or Motrin. Ashley had a headache because there was a disconnection—a hidden diagnosis—in the wires between her brain and a part of her body. *The exciting news is that within five minutes of my rehabilitation technique, the excruciating pain had completely subsided. The look on her face said more than any words I could write here.* I live for those moments, and that's why I decided to write about this new way of healing our bodies.   I'm sure you've experienced the sheer amount of medical advice floating around on TV, on the Internet, and on bookshelves in drugstores, doctors' offices, and even gas stations. Your local bookstore likely has aisles upon aisles of titles like these: *The one-week miracle cure for diabetes. The ancient headache healing plant. One-hundred ways to improve your memory. Seventy-five ways to feel better and live longer. Ten secrets to antiaging. Twenty-three ways to fight headaches.*

In many of these books, you'll find valuable advice for keeping certain parts of your body healthy, but the human body is a multi-faceted puzzle, one whose constituent parts work together intricately and inextricably. You can't separate out the various strands of the body's inner workings without neglecting other, important factors. Most of the books we find on bookstore shelves leave out comprehensive solutions to our underlying problems. In fact, many of them *just explain the problems* or provide temporary solutions that look myopically at one symptom of a larger dysfunction. With conventional healthcare, we have been programmed not to believe in the human machine. We don't believe that the body can fix itself. We don't think that it can heal itself *by* itself. Indefinite medicating is not the answer. Again, instead of fixing the problem, conventional healthcare centers on trying to fix symptoms of the problem.

We all like affirmations that we're not alone in our aches and pains, but why don't we begin to take back some responsibility for whole-body health? This book will outline a comprehensive plan for how to take care of your body, how to give your body the highest quality of life for the longest time possible. But you have to do your part. This book is no miracle cure, just a miraculous new way of looking at our amazing human body—through the lens of the nervous system. Miracle pills and spot treatments just don't exist. In order to achieve our best quality of life, we actually have to get off our butts and do the right things; we must look at your whole body health versus targeting specific ailments. Like everyone who embarks on a journey of self-improvement, whether it be athletically, spiritually, or emotionally, following the guidance of someone with firsthand experience is going to ensure that you take the most efficient steps to your goal. Doctors who have studied Quantum Neurology®, the concepts of which we'll discuss in depth in this book, particularly in Chapter 4, have the best comprehensive plan that's ever been invented for making the human body enjoy the highest quality of life regardless of who you are, what age you are, or what past experiences you've had. Quantum Neurologists are the masters of finding your hidden diagnosis and resolving it. The hidden diagnosis is a weak connection between your brain and one or more of your body parts. This book will give you the best explanation for why the human body does what it does and how to repair your body so that it's not going to break down as much as you've grown accustomed to.

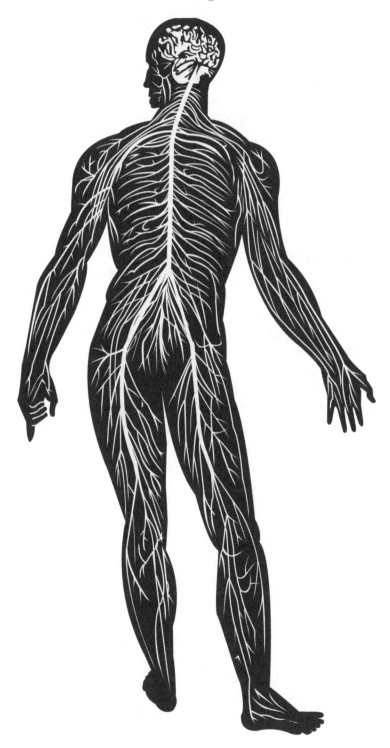

Why does anything I say matter? Of the slews of health and wellness books out there, why read mine? What I hope is that I can share my journey with you, the ways in which I've evolved my thinking over the years, and the common sense conclusions I've arrived at—and that you'll see the ways small lifestyle shifts can literally change your whole life. What I hope is that you'll see how I began my journey with a motivation to help my family members, from my dad to my wife and finally to my kids, seeking answers so that my loved ones wouldn't suffer. I developed this plan out of necessity; it's that very mother of invention that I want to share with you.

The way my wife and I, and by extension our kids, live our lives is totally different from the average American household. We aren't perfect. Our daily diet isn't perfect. But at the end of every day, we have given our bodies high-quality fuel additives and the best nervous system rehabilitation ever invented. The combination of the two keeps our bodies in check and allows us to function at peak levels without other types of interventions. We don't use over-the-counter stuff for headaches or colds. We use medicine only when it is absolutely necessary (as with a high fever), which is hardly ever. I'm not so arrogant as to believe that there won't be a time when traditional medicine is needed, but putting synthetic drugs into your system should be something that you only do when it's absolutely necessary. I'm not telling anyone to not use medicine. I'm telling everyone, however, that it's possible to use traditional medicine as a secondary instead of primary line of defense for a healthy life.

The secret to longevity involves a comprehensive plan that combines revolutionary thinking, good fuel, and expert nerve repair. We have to change the way we think and live accordingly before any significant changes happen to our collective health— and it's possible. Many animals can sense bad weather before it arrives. Humans have evolved to be savvy city dwellers, navigating people, confusing streets, and traffic jams. But when it comes to our bodies, we've checked out. Our bodies are innately intelligent; they know what they need, but most of us have forgotten how to listen. I'm about to tell you how my family lives and thrives, but first please remember this: you are the sole owner of the most amazing machine in existence, and you have your own model. It's your job to take care of this machine so you can do what you were called to do in this life. So, clear your bookshelves! When you're finished with this book, you'll have all the tools you'll need to get started. Change your thinking, and change your life.

PART I

Fueling the
Brain-to-Body
Connection

Patient Testimonial: *Al Broussard*

Since I was 17, I've had Parsonage-Turner syndrome, which affects the nerves. For a long time, I could barely put my arm over my head. Someone told me about Dr. C, and I went to him. He did some diagnostic testing on me and told me that I had a bundle of wrecked nerves. He was excited about that and said he could help me. By the time I went to him, my left bicep was gone, so he started working on it. I stuck with him for about three years and steadily improved. Now I can easily put my right arm over my head. I have strength back in my upper body. My left bicep returned. I love to fish. Before I went to Dr. C, after I fished for several hours, I could hardly move my wrist, and that's mostly diminished. I can live with that! The thing about Dr. C is if he can help you, he will. If he can't, he won't waste your time. He's always on the cutting edge of things—I was getting kind of bald, and he even made my hair grow back a little thicker. I go to Dr. C as often as I can for general well-being. He just makes me feel so much better. He doesn't put you on drugs or anything. Every time I go to the office, he's using something new. Vertical vibration, laser lights. It's amazing to watch. He loves his work.

Introduction: *The Marathon Brain*

The brain should be capable of running a marathon. Figuratively, our brains really should be in that kind of shape! A brain in marathon shape, with all of its nerves conditioned properly, equals a healthy body. Unfortunately, most people who come through my door are the folks who range from not very good brain function to terrible function because of the factors in their genetics and in their environments that hinder optimal nerve health. In the pages of this book, you'll begin to understand brain function and connectivity.

There are some people whose brains I'm just not able to get to 26.2 miles…yet. With Quantum Neurology's current level of technology, I can get them to 21 or 22 miles—these are the people who motivate me most to find new techniques. Everyone can achieve optimum health by maintaining a healthy nervous system. Because of the amazing things we're doing with nerve health techniques and body fueling systems, and because of the collaborative efforts of the handful of doctors practicing Quantum Neurology®, we're on the path to taking even the one-mile brain runners all the way to the finish line. We owe it to our bodies to take care of them as well as humanly possible—time and time again traditional thought has failed. I'm advocating a combination of small lifestyle changes, whole food supplements, and Quantum Neurology® for optimal nerve health. It's time for a revolution in the way we think about our health—our bodies can heal themselves, we just need to know how to aid the process.

Dr. Chris Cormier

Chapter 1: *The Journey*

In early 2007, my parents called my siblings and I and all of our spouses together for a sit-down meeting to discuss my father's health. It was a somber meeting—to say the least. My mother informed us that my 54-year-old dad had been placed on "The List" at Oschner's Hospital in New Orleans for a pancreas and kidney transplant. My father's kidney function had been barely above ten percent and his diabetes was out of control with blood sugar levels consistently greater than 200 (a normal blood sugar range is 90–120) despite taking insulin and other medications. His kidneys weren't far from failure, and dialysis was inevitable if a suitable donor couldn't be found. To top it all off, my dad vehemently refused to accept a kidney from a family member. We had finally reached the absolute lowest point of my dad's health.

This hadn't happened overnight. For more than two years, my father's feet were swollen so badly that they looked malformed. He was weak, at times barely able to walk. In fact, during our Thanksgiving meal in 2006, my dad got up from the table, but his legs were so weak that he tripped and fell hard enough that we took him to the emergency room. His overall demeanor was terrible—he slept on the couch for most of our family gatherings, couldn't interact with his beloved eight grandchildren.

In January 2007, he had a small stroke with a short period of slurred speech and partial paralysis of the left side of his body. This involved a long stay in the hospital. During his time in the hospital, my dad's blood sugar levels shot up to 400—with constant monitoring, despite taking insulin and other prescription medications for diabetes. Long-term high blood sugar, or hyperglycemia, causes a plethora of dangerous events to occur in the human body. High concentrations of sugar in the blood make it thick and syrupy, and the body has to fight to circulate it. Eventually, people suffering with this condition end up with problems like detached retinas, kidney failure, and multiple other organ failures. Polyneuropathy, or degeneration of the nerves, can take over, especially in the arms and legs, causing many patients to lose the ability to walk, feel their feet, and perform normal tasks like opening a jar. My dad was experiencing major symptoms of polyneuropathy, including noticeable indentations where the muscles in his hands had atrophied.

When my dad was diagnosed with diabetes in 1988, he tried to be diligent about making changes to his lifestyle but diet and exercise fell by the wayside after a few years. My dad's true passion had always been rice and soybean farming, a job that afforded him lots of physical activity and good meals every night on a regular schedule, but in 1991 he chose to change careers mainly due to low commodity prices. His new job was truck driving and dispatching for an oil company. This drastic lifestyle change included late-night truck stop fare, lots of caffeine-loaded fountain drinks, and a dire lack of exercise. Couple those with 30 years of smoking and you have a recipe for terrible health.

As a practicing chiropractic physician, I had tried everything to help my dad up to this point: chiropractic treatments, nutritional products, medical doctors, all to no avail. My dad had every natural and medical test and treatment imaginable, but his health was rapidly declining despite taking numerous supplements and thirteen prescription medications each day. He'd had multiple MRIs, CTs, biopsies, bone scans, and blood tests. Friends and colleagues (neurologists, neurosurgeons, radiologists, endocrinologists, etc.) had tried to help, but my dad was dying despite their efforts. These are the pivotal points in our lives—when the people we love are in pain, sick, or dying. I believed I could find a way to help him.

Thus began my journey into the world of nutrition and nerve rehabilitation, though the story may actually begin even before I was born when my Cajun ancestors were exiled from their homeland in Nova Scotia during the French and Indian War in the mid-18th century. They were literally dropped off by ship in the southern part of Louisiana, literally deported from their homeland. Many of these Cajuns died during this ordeal some who survived built a Cajun culture rich in music, religion, cuisine, and language. I think our cultural heritage is important to who we are. My great, great grandfather was not only a farmer, like so many of his neighbors, but also what Cajun people call a *traiteur* and a medicine man. My grandfather tells a story about suffering from terrible diarrhea as a child. His grandfather, the medicine man, went out into the woods, found a specific type of root, boiled the root, and fed the extract to my grandfather, who got better within several hours. His knowledge of prayer combined with whole foods and natural remedies helped many people in our region with their ailments. Modern medicine has moved away from roots and salves, but there are still plenty of people with the curiosity and drive to find real answers. In my case, I claimed my traiteur-and-medicine-man heritage in the brain-body connection.

There were probably four distinct events in youth childhood that set me on my particular path. In November 1982, when I was almost ten, my uncle was driving home from work when he was hit by a drunk driver. He was in a waking coma for the next ten years and died of pneumonia never having recovered brain function. We visited him in the hospital quite a bit. I remember how my uncle's eyes were open and moving around in his head, how he'd mumble on occasion. These visits were sobering for me but also, in a way, testified to the resilience of the human body that it could live after such a trauma. I remember—at 15, 16, 17 years old—thinking that there just had to be a way to help accident victims like my uncle.

When I was 11, my sister and I were sitting on her bed playing. Out of nowhere, her eyes rolled back in her head. She had a seizure, replete with major convulsions, right in front of me. In the end, my sister was fine, and it never happened again, but the image of something going terribly wrong in my sister's brain was brandished into my memory banks. In both instances, my uncle's crash from which he never recovered and my sister's one-time seizure, I knew there had to be answers.

When I got into Louisiana State University, I knew I was going to go into healthcare, but I wasn't quite sure which direction I'd take. At LSU, I majored in kinesiology and worked in hospitals as an aide whenever I could. I sat in on surgeries.

There were two instances, in particular, that made me realize I didn't want to go into traditional medicine. One summer, I was working in a surgery unit, and a sixty-eight-year-old retired medical doctor came in for surgery with gangrene in his foot. He was diabetic with polyneuropathy and had been walking out in his garden barefoot—which is a no-no for diabetics—when he cut his foot. The next thing you know, he had developed gangrene. By the time he came to the hospital for surgery, you could literally see through his foot. I'll never forget the smell of that gangrenous foot. During the surgery, I helped with the above-the-knee amputation—I was in charge of holding the bag into which the amputated lower leg was put. I just knew I didn't want to be part of this kind of solution. I wanted to help solve the problem.

The fourth experience involved a man who was having neck surgery. He was put into what's called a halo for surgery. Basically, his head was screwed into place and secured with metal bars so that his neck wouldn't move during and after surgery. When he was in post-op coming off anesthesia, he just went crazy. It took ten people to hold this guy down; he was throwing fists, pushing people, raging. They had to re-sedate him and bring him back into surgery because he'd torn something in his rage. Something about the violence of the experience, the way this man had to experience surgery, just felt wrong to me.

Through those college years, I worked with stroke victims, car accident victims, injuries of all sorts, and I got a wealth of experience. When I really looked at the traditional options, I saw that patients weren't dramatically improving. I don't know that I was ever fully invested in going the traditional route, but when my roommate became interested in chiropractic school, my curiosity was piqued.

Without ever having been to a chiropractor, I entered Texas Chiropractic College in Houston, where I became a member of the Omega Psi Honors Fraternity and received my Doctorate of Chiropractic with honors in 1998. Lucky for me, once I saw what the profession was all about, I thought, *I'm all in.*

Chiropractic care was a much more natural approach to dealing with the human body than the synthetics and cutting I had seen in hospitals. Chiropractors were trying to manage the body with resources the body already possesses, to find misalignments in the spinal bones. When normal alignment is restored to the spinal bones, pressure on the nerves gets alleviated. That just fell right in line with what I believed. Since then, I have been a licensed Chiropractic Physician in Louisiana and a member of the Chiropractic Association of Louisiana. I am also an affiliate of the American Chiropractic Association.

I started practicing in January of 1999, work five days a week in my practice, and see hundreds of patients every month. I specialize in treatment of the neuromusculoskeletal system, with a special interest in the healing power of nutrition. I have what I believe to be the absolute best technologies that the world has to offer for helping my patients—from infrared light to zero point energy. My patients feel comfortable asking my advice on all types of health conditions, trusting that if I can't help them, I will steer them to the correct specialist.

In my practice, I have taken a special interest in nutrition and whole food supplements because it is no secret that people who are better nourished each day have a much better quality of life. I am always searching for better ways to make people feel better. Better whole foods, better technologies, better treatments, better exercises, better posture—these are the things that I obsessively think about and are the basis for the lifestyle guidelines outlined in this book. I am committed to finding and implementing the best of everything in my practice, so my treatment is constantly evolving.

Chapter 2: *Fueling Your Body*

In a Youtube video called "The Power of Words," a blind man sits in front of a set of old church steps on a flattened out cardboard box. Next to him a sign reads, "I'm blind. Please help," but only a few people walking by hurriedly throw coins into his jar. All around him life goes on, and he goes virtually unnoticed. Then, a woman in a sleek business suit walks by him and doubles back. Without a word, she takes his sign and writes something different on the back of it. Suddenly, everyone who walks by is giving him change. When the businesswoman returns, presumably after her workday, she stops again to see the fruits of her labor, and the blind man asks, "What did you do to my sign?" and she replies, "I wrote the same but in different words." When the camera pans down, we see that the woman had written, "It's a beautiful day, and I can't see it."

We all want the same thing. We want to be healthy and happy. We want to provide for our families. But like the blind man in the video, we're not always going about it in the most effective way. We need to learn not just a *system*—there are so many systems already: weight loss, exercise, diets—but a new way of *thinking*, a new way of seeing the world.

Think about it this way. What has your body been exposed to since you were born? From stings to strokes, from teeth problems to broken bones, our bodies fight an uphill battle. We contend with colds, bacteria, and even cancer; we get into car accidents and recover from surgeries. We're stressed out daily by jobs, relationships, traffic jams. We eat prepackaged, processed foods and far too much. We drink too much alcohol, smoke cigarettes, abuse drugs. We suffer from neurological diseases, psychological diseases, skin diseases, lung diseases. We live in a world of pesticides and pollutants. We take prescription drugs to mask our symptoms. Really, in light of this, our daily lives are a testament to the power and resilience of the human body.

Pretend for a minute that your body is a car that you have been using and abusing since the day you were born. If you have incredible genetics and you've limited the abuse on your body, maybe you're a sleek Lamborghini. Or maybe you have less-than-perfect genetics; maybe you haven't taken care of yourself all that well and you're a run-down Yugo. Is your exterior terribly rusty? Is your upholstery torn and scratched up? Have you given your car its proper repairs? Have you gotten necessary oil changes? Tune-ups? Tire rotations? Filter Changes? Fixed scratches and dents? Have you given your car high-quality fuel, super octane with fuel additives, or the cheapest, dirtiest gas? Have you used carburetor or fuel injector cleaners? Are you getting the picture? *Why on earth don't we take care of our bodies the way we take care of our cars?*

If you want to run at optimum performance, you have to do the legwork to get there. You must properly fuel and repair every day, allowing your body's parts to efficiently function longer, which will ultimately give you a longer lifespan with a higher quality of life—even if you are predisposed to genetic diseases and malfunctions.

Humans haven't created anything as sophisticated or advanced as our own bodies. Chances are, you have probably taken it for granted. You have bills to pay, kids to raise, parents to care for. Instead of spending your time focused on your most valuable possession, you have focused on other things like fancy computers, cars, or your new Energy Star refrigerator. Like most of us, you likely haven't been listening to your body. If your car starts making a terrible clunking sound as you drive down the highway, what do you do? You get it fixed! The same should go for your body. When your body isn't running correctly, it will give you signs and symptoms like pain, numbness, tingling, cramping, dizziness, indigestion, bloating, irritability, constipation, weakness, fatigue, mood swings, burning, throbbing. Your body knows when something is wrong, and believe it or not, symptoms and pain are good. Your body gives you symptoms to alarm you that some wire has lost proper connectivity to your brain.

The most amazing thing about the human body is that it is a machine that, when properly wired, can heal itself of anything. You don't need spare parts or dealerships when it comes to your body because you already have the tools and parts you need to fix it. I even believe that there's already a cure for cancer. When your body is working on all cylinders, there's nothing it can't fix. The World Health Organization claims that nearly 40 percent of the cases of cancer can be prevented if people avoid the use of tobacco, carcinogens, and alcohol, and become physically active by doing exercise on a regular basis. How many people fight cancer on their own by changing their lifestyles? It's not just cancer, of course. Our bodies can heal arthritis, diabetes, heart disease, neuropathy, kidney disease, AIDS, lung diseases, digestive diseases, attention deficit. You name it. We are dynamic machines, constantly evolving to improve our functionality—everything from digestion to immunity to circulation of blood, making new blood cells, and repairing all damaged parts.

The human body instantly knows how to extrapolate nutrients from all the crazy foods we eat and gets rid of stuff it can't use. It has to stay on guard at all times, fully prepared to fight and win against all bad pathogens: viruses, bacteria, fungus, and parasites. For example, there's always some airborne fungus in the air we breathe. You can't go without breathing, so you're going to ingest spores. The reason those spores exist in the first place is because they're looking for a host on which to feed, so if you breathe in a bunch of these spores every day, your body has to be immediately on the defensive, differentiating between the good and bad fungal spores. Your brain has to decide on a dime whether or not to kill those spores. Occasionally, the brain will misunderstand what it's supposed to do, and this creates infection, whether sinus-related, bronchial, or tracheal. The spores will remain and cause allergies. The food we eat, particularly processed food, sits in warehouses, gets shipped all over the world, and oftentimes has pathogens on it. Our bodies have to be constantly vigilant for both the good and the bad in that processed food. The more processed food we eat, however, the harder the body has to work and the more likely it will be to make mistakes about what it needs and what it doesn't. As you'll see, we have to first change the way we think about taking care of ourselves before we can most effectively aid our bodies in that decision-making process.

Take Your Lab-Made Vitamins?

When I first started practicing, I'd order x-rays for people to get an idea of what was going on in their backs and spines. I consistently saw vitamin-shaped tablets on the x-rays, in the sigmoid colon, transverse colon, and descending colon—places where things are on their way out—which means that the body never even assimilated those vitamins. I have always taken great pride in recommending the best nutritional products for my patients, and the more undigested pills I saw in x-rays, the more nervous I got about recommending vitamin pills. Think about it. If you stick a bunch of synthetics in your body—if it's not a food that grows out of the earth—your body doesn't know what to do with it.

Most of the thirteen vitamins were discovered in the early twentieth century, when scientists found that diseases such as scurvy, rickets, and pellagra were caused by deficiencies of these essential substances. In the 1930s, we decided to take the vitamin C out of an orange, make it in a laboratory, and then give it to people in high dosages. vitamin C was the first vitamin to be synthesized and opened the floodgates for the vitamin revolution. Certainly vitamins must have seemed like the answer to nutritional deficiencies. Now, millions of people take high dosages of synthetic vitamin C every day. How is it that we came to believe that taking this laboratory-made vitamin C could be better than eating an orange? Well, there was a time when oranges weren't readily available to everyone, that's how. Vitamins are simply an imperfect step on the ladder of nutritional understanding.

Did you know that despite all of our country's superior technology, our leading scientists still don't know all of the ingredients and their average ratios in something as simple as an orange, apple, or pear? The nutrients in naturally grown whole foods, like oranges, are preassembled by nature in ratios that we are simply incapable of duplicating in a laboratory. Nature honors balance, not potency, and whole foods have the perfect ratio of vitamins, bioflavonoids, trace minerals, and all nutritional components working in perfect harmony. If you see specific amounts of vitamins added to a supplement, it is often because synthetically isolated (usually chemical) compounds are added in "one amount fits all" quantities. The reality is that one amount can't possibly fit all since we all have varied needs based on our age, health, lifestyle, and family history.

By the mid-twentieth century, a new generation of scientists began to dispute the value of vitamin supplements. This was not a debate about the importance of vitamins, since everyone agrees they are essential. Instead, the issue became whether or not lab-made vitamin supplements added to overall wellness. The skeptics rightly pointed out that only tiny amounts of vitamins are needed to prevent deficiency diseases. In the U.S. and other industrial societies, economic progress and improved nutrition have virtually eliminated vitamin-deficiency diseases. If a balanced diet can do the trick, why pop vitamin pills? The debate was on.

When you look on a vitamin bottle label, you see a list of individual vitamins and their respective dosages. The vitamin manufacturers take some of the individual vitamin properties that you find in grown foods, heighten the amounts, and load you with individual vitamins that your body can't assimilate. Your body, in turn, gets rid of things it can't process. The body likes the vitamins in naturally grown whole foods—that's the way the body is programmed to assimilate nutrients. The ingredients listed on the label of your daily supplement should list naturally grown whole foods like apples, pears, and peaches, for example, instead of vitamins like vitamins A, B, C, D, E and elements like calcium, magnesium, and zinc.

Think about it in the same way you think about fuel for your car. When you buy your car, the instruction manual tells you specifically what type of fuel you should use: diesel, 87 octane-rated gasoline, 88 octane-rated gasoline, 89 octane-rated gasoline, and so on. If there were an instruction manual for the human body, the fuel instructions would read the following: whole, organically grown fruits, vegetables, and grains.

Here are the reasons whole foods are the best fuel for our bodies:

Whole foods give our bodies nutrients that are already preassembled and prepackaged for proper digestion and ultimately give the body immediate, ready-to-use, fuel for daily activities.

Whole foods have hundreds, maybe thousands, of vitamins, minerals, phytonutrients, amino acids, and enzymes.

"Whole foods" should equate to "all natural," which means "derived directly from nature."

In rethinking the efficacy of pill-form vitamins and discovering the beauty of whole foods, I questioned whether or not whole foods could be taken in capsules, pills, or powders. I found a few companies with great all-whole-food products but didn't want to recommend that patients buy five, ten, or fifteen bottles of the different whole foods they'd need, things like aloe vera capsules, Pau d'Arco capsules, sea vegetable capsules (seven different types), açai berry powder or capsules, and on and on and on. It just wasn't practical or cost effective for patients to buy all these whole food supplements. The simple fact was that it was a challenge to patients to consistently take even one supplement per day, let alone a cabinet full.

Antioxidants and Free Radicals

Your body is made up of several trillion cells, each of which has a specific function and responsibility, and each of which needs high-quality fuel every day in order to accomplish all of its daily tasks and to keep brain-to-body nerve connections strong. The several trillion cells in your body labor like ants in a colony. Each individual ant may be tiny and may not move very quickly by our standards, but each has its specific responsibility to help maintain the entire colony or the colony's well-being is jeopardized. Likewise, if even one cell isn't fueled properly, your body won't run as efficiently as it should. Years of inadequate nutrition, along with the wear-and-tear of other stressors, can cause damage, which means that hundreds, thousands, millions, or even trillions of your body's cells are not functioning properly, causing the physical signs of aging that we are all too familiar with: dry skin, brittle hair, slowed metabolism and hormone production, fatty deposits, slowed gait, lack of coordination, hearing loss, visual problems. If you combine a sustained poor diet with other daily stressors of the average American, you have a recipe for disaster.

In the process of breaking down and metabolizing food, getting air in and out of our cells, and as bi-products of the immune system's battles with colds, other viruses, bacteria, or other diseases, the cells in our bodies produce trash which is called free radicals. These free radicals are also produced as a result of exposure to pollution like cigarette smoke or car exhaust. Antioxidants, like those from colorful super berries, for instance, mop up these destructive free radicals.

It is well known that most Americans do not eat enough antioxidant rich foods at each meal, leading to excessive trash (free radical) build-up around our cells, which ultimately damages DNA and cell membranes in a process called oxidative stress. This whole scenario creates a more favorable environment for diseases like atherosclerosis and cancer to flourish. As you might imagine, when cells are less efficient, brain-to-body connectivity is more susceptible to weakness.

Every day for over fifty years, many Americans have eaten an average combination of the following:

- Fewer than two grocery-bought fruits
- Fewer than three grocery-bought vegetables
- Processed foods and liquids
- Maybe a couple of synthetic laboratory-made vitamins or supplements

The majority of our diets consist of processed foods: anything canned, packaged, frozen, or bagged has been processed. We rarely eat anything directly from the farm to our mouths, and even more rarely do we eat organic farm food. Most of what we eat is from a laboratory or manufacturing facility. Processed foods are supersaturated with preservatives and additives that hinder our brains' functionality. We are conditioned to eat poorly, and we've become addicted to bad diets. We're inundated by fast food burgers and delicious blended coffee drinks, greasy potato chips, all-day soft drinks in refillable 20 ounce cups, so how on earth can we eat perfectly every day in order to fuel our bodies optimally? We'll sometimes eat processed foods. All we can do is try to eat whole foods whenever humanly possible and cook our own food at home with real vegetables and fruits and organic meats.

Taken a step further, I recommend the personalized GenoType Diets™, which is a revolutionized version of the *Eat Right for Your Type* diet. Naturopathic physician Peter D'Adamo, author of *Eat Right for Your Type,* recently published a new book called *Change Your Genetic Destiny: The Revolutionary GenoType Diet* whereby he expands his approach to diet and health beyond the four blood types by profiling six "GenoTypes." According to Dr. D'Adamo, tailoring diet and lifestyle to GenoTypes (genetic survival strategies that predate ethnicity and race and correspond to such external traits as body type, jaw shape, and teeth patterns) is the most effective way to achieve optimum health. This diet takes into account everything from your blood type, to your personal family and medical history, to personality traits, to body measurements. Let's be realistic. I have children, and my children sometimes eat Pop-Tarts for breakfast. This is the state of modernity. The antidote is to try to eat well for your personalized GenoType and to take a fuel additive each day that contains a liquid mixture of the right fuel. I know I'm not going to convince everyone to totally stop eating junk food, so what I'm advocating is balance and a solid understanding of the best foods for your body.

The Pathogen Problem: *Consuming GMOs*

These days, it's hard to achieve balance in our diets, but the best way is to eat organic foods. Having spent my childhood and teen years on a farm, I know a thing or two about farming practices, and I've seen how farming has changed over the span of my own lifetime. As a student of nutrition, I have come to understand how eating non-organic foods can affect our brain-to-body connections.

Our world consists of four main pathogens: fungus, bacteria, parasites, and viruses. Many of these are harmless, and even beneficial, to the body. But, the body has to be able to recognize what's good and what's bad as it's ingesting and encountering all of these pathogens.

The problem is this: human intervention into natural processes has sped up the evolution of pathogens by a thousand years. Super fungus drugs like antibiotics have caused bacteria to morph into super-bacteria. I'm not saying antibiotics are bad—I'm saying that overutilization of antibiotics has created a massive problem. Antibiotics are mold (a fungus), one of the subcategories of pathogens, and fungus (specifically mold) in nature is always at war with bacteria. Scientists have recently shown that a fungus decimating amphibian populations all over the globe has a natural enemy in the bacteria found on the skin of several different salamander species.[1]

In the human body, the pharmaceutical companies started using fungus to battle bacteria. A great idea, but we started using too much. Bacteria started mutating, becoming stronger and stronger, and in laboratories we tried to keep up, fabricating stronger antibiotics. In a microscopic keeping-up-with-the-Joneses scenario, fungi have responded to these super-bacteria by morphing into bigger and better species. As a result, there is too much fungus in our bodies, speeding up the evolution of fungus and bacteria. This is why you hear crazy stories about

---

[1] Anitei, Stefan. "Bacteria Found to Fight Killer Fungus," *Softpedia*, May 2007. http://news.softpedia.com/news/Bacteria-Found-to-Fight-the-Killer-Fungus-56003.shtml)

bacteria that didn't exist before (such as flesh-eating bacteria). The evolution of pathogens is occurring so quickly that our immune systems are under enormous pressure to keep up.

Our Food Sources

This kind of accelerated evolution has also happened with all our food sources in crops grown throughout the world. Because we need more crops—and quickly—for our growing populations, in an effort to speed up the harvesting process as well as garner control of the unwelcome plants and insects living amidst and feasting on our crops, we now have chemicals to take care of the invaders.

On the farm where I grew up, we planted rice. Every season we would get a weed in the rice that we call "red rice." Red rice actually degrades your rice in harvest by reducing its worth. When I was a kid, I used to go out into the fields and hand pull the red rice from the fields. Although it was very labor intensive, at that time it was the best way to get rid of the weeds so that, when harvested, the value of the crop wouldn't go down. The same for soybeans: we had what we called indigos that grew amidst the crop. We'd uproot the indigos with our bare hands to ensure maximum yield of soy. Today, in an effort to stop endless hours of manual labor, there are chemicals on the market strong enough that when sprayed on the field, *everything* will die but the crop you're growing.

I don't know if a light bulb just went off in your head, but it should have. Spraying a chemical that kills everything else but the specific crop you're trying to harvest means that some change has occurred with that crop. Corn seed, for instance, is being genetically modified to resist certain chemicals, namely those made to kill the invasive species. So, as a farmer, you buy the genetically modified seeds (GMOs), knowing that you'll spray the whole field, kill the stuff you don't want, and keep the good crop—without having to use the manpower to pull the weeds. It sounds great in theory, but when you start feeding livestock and humans GMO grains, we've all got major problems.

If you kill everything in that field except your crop, what do you think is growing in the periphery of that field? The killed-off weeds grow back elsewhere with a vengeance, mutating so they are more difficult to kill the next time. The chemical manufacturers have realized this, altering and strengthening their chemicals every four or five years in order to keep up with the pace of evolution of pathogens that are in these fields. In turn, they continue to genetically modify seeds to be resistant to these new chemical blends. This is a major compound problem, and literally trickles into our bodies through the crops themselves and the livestock eating them. With the way our country is progressing, it won't be long before all seeds, grains, and foods are genetically modified. In fact, right now, almost all corn and soybeans are genetically modified—and it is virtually impossible to keep corn or soybean products out of your diet.

Because we are eating GMOs that our bodies really don't know how to process, our bodies, and the meat of the animals we eat, have become walking hotels for pathogens. In essence, in our human drive to create and improve, we've created a monster. Even our statin drugs for high cholesterol and many anticancer drugs are made out of fungi. While we're trying to use fungus to help the body, we're actually creating an imbalance of pathogens, which is why it is even more imperative to get the right fuel for your body every day.[2]

---

[2] "Genetically Engineered Food Alters Our Digestive Systems," *Alliance for Natural Health,* May 2011.http://www.anh-usa.org/genetically-engineered-food-alters-our-digestive-systems

Liquid Food Revolution:
The SeaAloe Discovery

Armed with the knowledge of poor eating habits, processed foods, pathogen-charged crops, and ineffective vitamins, I began researching other forms of whole foods. I started reading more and more information on whole food liquids and really liked what I was finding. Liquefying whole foods meant that the integrity of each whole food was maintained but reduced to tiny particles that were ready for immediate, full absorption in the small intestines of anyone—from five-year-olds to ninety-five-year-olds. Bottom line: I wanted something better for my patients and my family. In January 2002, I discovered the SeaAloe formula (formerly called Seasilver) and fell in love with its whole food liquid mixture that uses the highest quality naturally grown whole foods from the best sources in the world. I trust this product with my own family; hence, I'll use SeaAloe as an example of what we *should* be putting into our bodies and what you should look for in a liquid whole food product.

SeaAloe blends thirteen different whole foods, including seven different sea vegetables, aloe vera, Pau d'Arco, cranberry, white grape, Concord grape, and black cherry. SeaAloe contains nothing synthetic or laboratory made. Too many formulas try to get too fancy by adding unnecessary ingredients; SeaAloe keeps it simple with fewer, better quality ingredients. On the more scientific side, SeaAloe uses proprietary processing techniques that reduce surface tension to 25 percent below that of water for enhanced absorption and cellular bio-availability.

My family and I have taken the SeaAloe formula every day now for more than nine years, and I have never found anything more beneficial to energy and overall well-being on a daily basis. My wife used SeaAloe as a prenatal vitamin with all of her pregnancies, and my children have taken SeaAloe every single day of their lives—in fact, they ask for it morning and evening. Over 2000 studies have been conducted on sea vegetation and how sea vegetables help to normalize cellular health. They are perfectly suited for human biology.

It's so important to understand the products you put into your body. Sure, sea vegetables, aloe vera, and cranberry sound like they might have health benefits. But what does that really mean? How can an aloe plant do anything but alleviate sunburn pain? What on earth is a sea vegetable? I drink cranberry juice cocktail all the time; does that mean I'm getting all of the benefits a cranberry has to offer? Below is a list of SeaAloe's ingredients and why they are beneficial—apart from the fact that all the ingredients have been harvested and manufactured properly, which is essential for maximum benefit.

Aloe Vera

The use of aloe vera can be traced back six thousand years to ancient Egypt where the plant has been depicted on stone carvings. Known as the "plant of immortality," aloe was presented as a burial gift to deceased Egyptian pharaohs.

Today people take aloe orally to treat a variety of conditions, including diabetes, asthma, epilepsy, and osteoarthritis. People use aloe topically for osteoarthritis, burns, and sunburns. Aloe vera contains active compounds called glycoproteins, which may decrease low levels of pain and inflammation. Additionally, aloe vera contains polysaccharides, which have been shown to support skin regeneration and repair. Aloe vera is internally and topically beneficial, with stabilizing properties that can support normal blood sugar levels. Aloe vera has commonly been used for sunburn relief, and its moisture-like properties work the same externally as they do internally.

Currently, no adverse side effects have been reported from ingesting the inner gel of the aloe vera plant when it is properly processed. Aloe products should use hand-filleted aloe, cold processing, and only the plant's inner gel. If you see products that are machine-processed, whole leaf, dehydrated or pasteurized, stay away! You're not getting the health benefits you should.

Quick Reference: *What can aloe vera do for me?*

- Supports normal gastrointestinal function
- Cleanses the internal organs
- Provides powerful nutritional value
- Contains antifungal properties
- Contains anti-inflammatory properties

Sea Vegetables

Because of depleted nutrient values in soil due to industrial agriculture, we have recently had to turn to the ocean for nutrient rich, bio-available sources of quality supplementation. Additionally, sea-based nutrition thrives in a salt-water based environment, which is similar to the make-up of the human body (70–80 percent salt water). Sea vegetables are neither plants nor animals but classified in a group known as algae. There are thousands of types of sea vegetables, but a superior product contains only the varieties highest in nutritional value versus micro portions of thousands of vegetables. SeaAloe, for instance, uses (1)*Ascophyllum nodosum* (2) Kelp (3) *Fucus vesiculosus* (4) Fucus (5) Chondrus crispus (6) Nori (7) *Ulva lactuca* and procures its sea vegetables from the coldest and purest waters off Iceland and Canada.

Sea vegetables have been used in Eastern cultures for many thousands of years. Archaeological evidence suggests that Japanese cultures have been consuming sea vegetables for more than 10,000 years. As early as 100 B.C., the Greeks collected seaweed. Since pre-Christian times all along the Mediterranean coast, red alga has been used as a medicine to treat parasitic worms. In fact, most regions and countries located by waters, including Scotland, Ireland, Norway, Iceland, New Zealand, the Pacific Islands, and coastal South American countries have been consuming sea vegetables since ancient times.

Sea vegetables also been used for their antiviral effects and support of normal adrenal functions. An abundant source of vitamins and minerals, sea vegetables effectively support normal immune system functions. Sea vegetables also contain high levels of protein and amino acids, which are essential for cellular division. Sea vegetables also contain organic (photosynthetic) vitamins, trace minerals, lipids, plant sterols, amino acids, omega-3, omega-6, antioxidants, growth hormones, polyphenols, and flavonoids. They also contain powerful fucoidan, laminarin, and alginate compounds, which studies suggest are antibiotic and antiviral. These phytochemicals are not found in land plants. Sea vegetables are the richest natural source of minerals, trace minerals and rare earth elements.

Quick Reference: *What can sea vegetables do for me?*

- Contain sources of heart-protective magnesium, potassium, and beta-carotene
- Support normal thyroid functions
- Are excellent sources of highly absorbable plant-based calcium
- Are concentrated sources of vitamins, minerals, and amino acids

Pau d'Arco

Pau d'Arco is extracted from the inner bark of the Tabebuia genus tree, which is found in South and Central America and, occasionally, Florida and has been used for thousands of years among indigenous tribes of South America to treat cancer, inflammation, and a host of other infections.

Pau d'Arco has also been studied to help increase the production of red blood cells, which carry the body's oxygen supply and remove carbon dioxide from the blood stream, and it possesses immunostimulating properties that help support normal immune system functions. Pau d'Arco should always be properly processed to release the volatile oils and esters for maximum effectiveness and strength. It should never be fumigated, irradiated, or contain excipients, binders, or fillers.

Quick Reference: *What can Pau d'Arco do for me?*

- Supports normal lymphatic system functions
- Antiviral properties
- Antibacterial properties
- Supports normal immune system functions
- Analgesic (painkilling) effects
- Helps maintain bowel regularity

4 Fruit Juice Blend: *Cranberries*

Cranberries are one of three (along with blueberries and Concord grapes) native North American fruits that are commercially grown. Native Americans used cranberries for their healing properties and as food. Today, cranberries are grown in multiple states in the U.S., primarily in Maine, Massachusetts, Michigan, Minnesota, New Jersey, Oregon, Washington, and Wisconsin. Cranberries belong to the evergreen family and typically fruit during the calendar months of June and July.

Recently, cranberries have been used in medical studies concerned with free radical management. Free radicals located in the brain have been shown to cause damage to motor and cognitive functions. Consumption of cranberries is currently being researched to evaluate their antioxidant benefits and how those antioxidants can fight free radicals in brain cells.

Quick Reference: *What can cranberries do for me?*

- Provides an excellent source of vitamin C
- Aids in the prevention of developing urinary tract infections
- Supports regular gastrointestinal functions
- Lowers the buildup of dental plaque
- High in antioxidants

4 Fruit Juice Blend:
White and Concord Grapes

Concord grapes are commonly grown in the Pacific Northwest and Eastern United States. They are purple in color and provide many different health benefits. White grapes originated from Europe and are native to the Mediterranean region and central Asia. White grapes can be grown in many climates but are ideally grown in moderate temperate zones. White grapes are easy to digest so they make a great option for babies and children in lieu of apple or pear juices. White grapes and Concord grapes both contain phytochemical compounds called resveratrol, which I'll discuss later. These compounds have been shown to aid in the stabilization of capillary walls, supporting circulation and blood flow. These natural compounds have also been shown to have cardioprotective properties for those who consume them.

Quick Reference: *What can white and Concord grapes do for me?*

- Support flexibility in arteries
- Support normal blood pressure
- Help lower cholesterol
- Easy to digest
- Contain polyphenol antioxidants
- Have antifungal properties
- Support collagen and elastin levels in your skin

4 Fruit Juice Blend: *Black Cherries*

Black cherries typically contain 17 antioxidants that include anthocyanins—flavonoids that have some of the strongest antioxidant effects of any plant compound—and melatonin. Maintaining normal melatonin levels helps with memory and learning. Black cherries are native to North America and commonly grown in Texas, Florida, Arizona, and New Mexico. All the fruit supplements you take should come from reliable North American sources, ensuring that they're the freshest available. Bioactivity is destroyed in over-processed fruits, and sugar-and-preservative additions take away from their health value.

Quick Reference: What can black cherries do for me?

- Anti-inflammatory properties
- Help lower uric acids levels in the body
- Contain anthocyanins
- Antibacterial properties
- Reduce oxidative stress
- Antioxidant rich

The Superfruits GT Story

When I discovered that most of the products on the market were totally unregulated and seldom actually provided the nutrients their labels claimed, I decided to make my own using strictly naturally grown foods. Again, liquid foods allow you to give your body the best fuel in the world regardless of your diet. My liquid foods contain blends of the world's most potent antioxidant and disease-fighting whole foods.

While the SeaAloe formula does a lot in terms of antioxidant power, the one major thing lacking is super berry antioxidants. Our lives are filled with so many factors that drain our antioxidants, some of which I've already touched on: daily stress, caffeine, alcohol, smoking, and limited intake of high antioxidant fruits. And as I've said, antioxidants get rid of trash (free radicals) in your body's several trillion cells. When your body fills up with trash its functionality spirals downward. It's like living in a house and throwing nothing away. Eventually you can't even move through the piles of newspapers and plastic bottles, old clothes and unused gadgets. You're a prisoner in your own home!

One of the most antioxidant-rich foods on the planet, included in Superfruits GT, is the açai berry from Brazil's Amazon jungle. Unfortunately, there are hundreds of so-called açai berry products that are actually nothing more than watered down açai berry filled with sugar—made by greedy manufacturers taking advantage of the public. I'm sure by now that you are one of the millions of Americans who have heard about açai berry's health benefits. It has been featured on many different television shows and news segments. Doctors and health experts across the globe are calling the açai berry one of the world's best whole foods. This is the good news.

The sad part of the açai berry story is this: If you've spent your hard-earned money on an açai product, you've likely been scammed. This is a major fault of the nutrition industry. Supplement manufacturers know that they're not being regulated, and they take advantage of the consumer by manufacturing the cheapest products and selling these products at exorbitant prices. This pads their pocketbooks and ultimately gives them a tremendous profit margin, but it doesn't do much for you and me.

How do they do this? Let's look more closely at açai. First, manufacturers understand that they can get low quality açai berry for next to nothing. Cheap açai berries come to the U.S. almost rotten. They have not been properly transported, and the nutrients have almost totally oxidized. Second, manufacturers know that they only need to have a tiny amount of an ingredient to list it on the label. There could literally be a drop of açai in a product to label it as an açai product. As you've probably guessed, there aren't many therapeutic benefits to one drop of anything. In addition, pure açai is bitter. If your açai product tastes sweet, you can be sure açai isn't its primary ingredient.

The ORAC score (Oxygen Radical Absorbance Capacity), or the amount of antioxidants present in your product, is also important to look at. The USDA (United States Department of Agriculture) has established ORAC scores for almost all whole foods (e.g., oranges, apples, pears). Simply put, the ORAC method measures a whole food's ability to clean up the trash around our cells and destructive free radicals like the "peroxyl radical" which is one of the most common free radicals found in the human body.

Because this is an emerging technology, there has not been much research done on the efficacy of high ORAC scoring foods and their effects on human health, but in the years to come there will certainly be extensive studies done to demonstrate the power of these high ORAC whole foods.

If your açai berry product does not have an ORAC score from an official testing facility (e.g., Brunswick Labs) on its label or its official website, then said product most likely does not have a good ORAC score, which means that the product does not contain a high level of antioxidants. Some açai berry products have validated ORAC scores that are high, but one must still be careful. Scamming occurs with these high ORAC products as well. Instead of loading a product with high amounts of antioxidant rich açai berries, manufacturers can trick the system by loading high amounts of laboratory prepared antioxidant vitamins like C or E.

The tragedy is that in the next five to ten years, Americans are going to start to believe that the açai berry really doesn't help them at all. All of this is because they have taken products with miniscule amounts of bad berries. Of course, açai berry is not the only superfood that this process happens with. This very same scamming process happens with many other world superfoods, such as mangosteen, pomegranate, goji berry, and blueberry.

In order to carefully manufacture a high-quality, low-price product that included whole foods like açai, it took my team over a year and a half to complete the Superfruits GT formula, which we released in 2009. Superfruits GT offers a blend of nine whole foods (açai berry, goji berry, mangosteen, pomegranate, blueberry, peach, pear, white grape, and green tea).

ORAC testing at the renowned Brunswick Laboratories showed Superfruits GT to have a total ORAC score of an astounding 1,750 per ounce. Just three ounces of Superfruits GT a day gives the body an amazing dosage of whole food antioxidants. Like SeaAloe, Superfruits GT uses an exclusive process that reduces surface tension to 25 percent below that of water for enhanced absorption and cellular bioavailability. Just one ounce of Superfruits GT has the exact same amount of resveratrol as over 100 glasses of red wine.

Resveratrol is a potent antioxidant that has been popular in the news lately. In January 2009, *60 Minutes* aired a special highlighting the research being conducted on resveratrol. The *60 Minutes* special referred to resveratrol as the long lost "Fountain of Youth."

Superfruits GT contains a natural source of resveratrol in a non-alcoholic form, making it accessible for almost everyone to take. Just one ounce of Superfruits GT has the same amount of antioxidants as over seven bananas.

How is this possible? How did a chiropractor from a small town in Southern Louisiana create such an incredible antioxidant product at double the strength for less than half the price of other products? Here's how:

a) We use FDA-approved high-density polyethylene (HDPE) bottles, which aren't as fancy as the expensive wine bottles or other odd-shaped glass bottles used by my competitors. This means less money spent on packaging and shipping and more money spent on actual ingredients. More money spent on ingredients means higher quantity of ingredients in our formula.

b) We have the best liquid manufacturer in the U.S., who has relationships with wholesale suppliers across the world that no one else has. He always gets the highest quality ingredients for lesser prices. He manufactures only our products so he's not overloaded and cutting corners.

c) Because we are so product focused, we are willing to accept a smaller profit margin in order to make the highest quality and highest quantity formula on the market. We still make money; we're just not in this for gouging the public.

I'll use the ingredients in Superfruits GT to outline the health benefits of the best, most trustworthy liquid fuel.

Açai Berries

We just talked about the dangers of trusting many açai products, but here's why it's so important to get *good* açai. Açai berries grow on an Amazon palm tree and look like a purple marble or a grape. In traditional Brazilian populations, the açai fruit makes up a huge portion of the daily diet. The "açai bowl," consisting of a cold-blended açai and other fruits and topped with granola, is a popular snack both in Brazil and in many parts of the United States, where it appears on breakfast menus and in smoothie bars.

Açai pulp contains 10–30 times the antioxidants of red wine per equal volume. Açai berries are rich in B vitamins, minerals (particularly iron in food-form), fiber, proteins, essential fatty acids, and anthocyanins. The ORAC value of açai berry is higher than any other edible berry on the planet. Açai berry is also an excellent source of dietary fiber, high in essential fatty acids, including omega-3 and omega-6 that have been found to support normal low levels of LDL & HDL cholesterol. Fatty acids also aid in the transport and absorption of fat-soluble vitamins such as A, E, D, and K.

Quick Reference: *What can açai berries do for me?*

- One of the highest level antioxidant berries on the planet
- Aid in antiaging
- Cardiovascular support
- Powerful nutritional value
- Normal cholesterol supporting properties
- Support normal immune system functions
- Studies currently being done on anti-cancer effects

Goji Berries

Goji are bright red berries native to Southeastern Europe and Asia. When ripe, the berries are collected by shaking the vines over special mats where they are untouched and left to dry under the Himalayan sun. It is vital that the berries are never touched by the human hands when they are fresh, otherwise they will oxidize, causing them to turn black and become unusable.

There is more beta-carotene in goji berries than in carrots, and they contain more vitamin C than oranges. They are also a rich source of naturally occurring B1, B2, B6, vitamin E, essential fatty acids, and polysaccharides. Goji berries have 18 amino acids (including eight essential amino acids.) Essential amino acids cannot be produced by the body and must come from the food we eat. Goji berries also contain trace minerals and protein.

Quick Reference: What can goji berries do for me?

- One of the highest level antioxidant berries on the planet
- Improve concentration
- Improve memory
- Aid in antiaging
- Support normal immune system functions
- Increase energy

Mangosteen

Contrary to popular belief, mangosteen is not a mango. It is a tropical fruit discovered in 1697. The inside portion of the berry is a pale, fleshy fruit. The primary plant growing area for the healthful mangosteen fruit is in Southeast Asia, and commercial growing of the mangosteen tree has been largely unsuccessful in other climates of the world. Mangosteen has been used for centuries in Southeast Asia to ward off infections and headaches, reduce pain and swelling, control fever, and various other ailments. Mangosteen has also been used for centuries in some countries for its strong anti-inflammatory and antihistamine properties.

In addition to its anti-inflammatory effects in numerous studies, mangosteen is rich in antioxidants, including powerful xanthones found in the outer rind (pericarp) of the fruit, which have been studied for their antitumor, antiproliferative, antimicrobial, antihistamine, anti-inflammatory, antioxidant, and gastrointestinal protective effects. The mangosteen also contains catechins, the antioxidants found in green tea.

Quick Reference: What can mangosteen do for me?

- Aids in antiaging
- Has anti-inflammatory properties
- Has antibacterial properties
- Supports normal immune system functions

Pomegranate

The name "pomegranate" comes from the Latin for seeded apple and is a prominent symbol in ancient myth and legend. Pomegranate is one of the earliest cultivated fruits and is native from Iran to the Himalayas in Northern India. The pomegranate has been cultivated and naturalized over the whole Mediterranean region and the Caucasus since ancient times.

The major antioxidants in pomegranate seeds are called punicalagins, which break down into ellagic acid. Pomegranate also contains other antioxidants such as vitamin C, beta-carotene, catechins, gallocatechins, and anthocyanins such as prodelphinidins, delphinidin, cyanidin, and pelargonidin. The ORAC (Oxygen Radical Absorbance Capacity) value of pomegranate juice is considered high, measured at approximately 10,500 units per 100 grams.

Quick Reference: What can pomegranate do for me?

- Aids in antiaging processes
- Has anti-inflammatory properties
- Is high in antioxidants

Blueberries

Blueberries are native to North America, with around thirty different species, and played an important role in North American Indian food culture, being an ingredient in pemmican, a traditional dish composed of fruit and dried meat. Blueberries weren't cultivated until the beginning of the twentieth century, however, available commercially beginning in 1916.

Based on data from the USDA Human Nutrition Research Center on Aging (Boston, MA), blueberries are among the fruits with the highest antioxidant activity. Researchers have shown that a serving of fresh blueberries provided more antioxidant activity than many other fresh fruits and vegetables. Just one cup of blueberries contains 14 milligrams of vitamin C and 0.8 milligrams vitamin E. In addition, blueberries contain anthocyanins and phenolics that can also act as antioxidants. Anthocyanin gives blueberries their color and might be the key component of the blueberry's antioxidant and anti-inflammatory properties. Blueberries, along with other colorful fruits and vegetables, test high in their ability to subdue free radicals.

Quick Reference: What can blueberries do for me?

- Aid in antiaging processes
- Have anti-inflammatory properties
- Contain anthocyanins
- Reduce oxidative stress
- Are antioxidant rich

Peaches

The Persian apple, as it was once known, hails from ancient China and is a symbol of longevity and mentioned in Chinese writings as far back as the 10th century B.C. In the 1600s, Spanish missionaries planted peach trees in America. Native Americans are credited with migrating the peach tree across the U.S., where they planted the seeds as they traveled. Today, California, South Carolina, and Georgia are the largest producers of peaches. The peach is considered the most sacred plant of the Chinese Taoist religion, and today the peach is customarily served at birthday celebrations in China as a symbol and hope of longevity.

A member of the rose family, the peach is not only low in calories (one cup, sliced, has just 60), it's also packed with potassium—a medium peach has 285 milligrams (about 5 percent of your recommended daily allowance). Potassium is essential for the body's cell function and for maintaining a balance of fluids and electrolytes, important for nerve signaling, muscle contraction, and metabolism. Peaches are also an excellent source of vitamins A and C and the cancer-fighting antioxidant beta-carotene. According to researchers at Texas Agricultural Experiment Station, peaches are a great source of antioxidants and other phytochemicals, antimicrobial activity, and tumor growth inhibition activity.

Quick Reference: *What can peaches do for me?*

- Boost metabolism
- Loaded with vitamins A and C
- Aid in muscle health

Pears

Evidence of pear cultivation can be traced back to ancient times, and there is even evidence of pear consumption all the way back to prehistoric times. For instance, pears have been cultivated in China for nearly 3,000 years, and there exist recipes for stewed and spiced pears dating back to ancient Rome. Pears are native to most coastal, mildly temperate regions of Western Europe, North Africa, and Asia.

Pears are a good source of vitamin C and copper; both antioxidant nutrients help protect cells in the body from oxygen-related damage due to free radicals. Pears are an excellent source of water-soluble fiber. They contain vitamins A, B1, B2, C, E, folic acid, and niacin. They are also rich in phosphorus and potassium, with lesser amounts of calcium, chlorine, iron, magnesium, sodium, and sulfur. Pears are very unlikely to trigger allergic reactions, so can be used in exclusion diets. They contain hydroxycinnamic acids, which also act as antioxidants.

Quick Reference: What can pears do for me?

- Boost energy
- Support normal cholesterol levels
- Antioxidant rich

Resveratrol (*Polygonum cuspidatum*)

Resveratrol is a naturally occurring, powerful antioxidant found primarily in grape skin and seeds. New studies show that resveratrol slows the onset of virtually all of the aging diseases: heart, arthritis, cancers, and Alzheimer's. Others have shown it does still more—repairs alcohol-damaged livers, slows bone loss (osteoporosis), boosts endurance, promotes hair growth, and re-energizes cells. When scientists added resveratrol to the diet of yeast, fruit flies, worms, and a species of fish, their life spans increased up to 70 percent, 29 percent, 24 percent, & 50 percent, respectively.

We obtain our resveratrol from Japanese knotweed (*Fallopia japonica*, syn. *Polygonum cuspidatum, Reynoutria japonica*), which is a large, herbaceous perennial plant, native to Eastern Asia in Japan, China and Korea. We selected this particular plant because it gives us a more consistent source of high quality resveratrol, growing year-round and resilient to all types of weather. Japanese knotweed is also extremely concentrated with high-grade resveratrol.

Quick Reference: *What can resveratrol do for me?*

- Increases energy
- Increases endurance
- Contains anthocyanins
- Currently being studied for its anticancer properties
- Maintains normal low levels of cholesterol
- Powerful antioxidant

Green Tea (*Camellia sinensis*)

Green tea was discovered over five thousand years ago. Legend has it that an emperor was drinking hot water when a tea leaf fell into his cup, and the rest is history. Green tea is made from the leaves of the *Camellia sinensis* plant that have undergone minimal oxidation.

Green tea is particularly rich in health-promoting flavonoids (which account for 30 percent of the dry weight of a leaf), including catechins and their derivatives. The most abundant catechin in green tea is epigallocatechin-3-gallate (EGCG), which plays a pivotal role in the green tea's anticancer and antioxidant effects. Catechins should be considered right alongside the better-known antioxidants like vitamins E and C as potent free radical scavengers.

Most research showing the health benefits of green tea is based on the amount of green tea typically consumed in Asian countries—about three cups per day. Green tea drinkers appear to have lower risk for a wide range of diseases, from simple bacterial or viral infections to chronic degenerative conditions, including cardiovascular disease, cancer, stroke, periodontal disease, and osteoporosis. The health benefits of green tea have been extensively researched and, as the scientific community's awareness of its potential benefits has increased, so have the number of new studies. As of 2008, the PubMed.com database contained more than 3,000 studies on green tea illustrating its numerous health benefits.

Quick Reference: *What can green tea do for me?*

- Increases energy
- Increases endurance
- Contains anthocyanins
- Studied for its anticancer properties
- Has powerful antioxidants called catechins

The Chiropractor's Choice Story

What I didn't understand at first as I was trying to find a cure for my father was that, neurologically speaking, before he could exercise at all as part of a healthy lifestyle, his body needed repair. His nervous system was functioning so badly that he was using all his energy just barely getting through each day. His brain was so poorly connected with the rest of his body that, by midday, his fuel tank was empty.

To start, I needed an anti-inflammatory product that would help get rid of the swelling in my dad's feet. Prescriptions were doing no good in this department, and none of the natural or vitamin products I tried with him were working either.

I needed something specific to chiropractic concerns for all of my patients as well, so I searched high and low for the world's most powerful superfoods with anti-inflammatory properties. During this process, I discovered some incredible whole foods that very few other products contained, but as I am particular about what I look for in a good anti-inflammatory product, I limited my search:

I wanted only the highest quality whole foods most beneficial for patients' main concerns: inflammation, pain, and arthritis.

I wanted to make this product available through chiropractors.

I wanted this product to give patients immediate therapeutic benefits. In other words, I didn't want to make a diluted, low dosage formula that would help our patients only after several months of use. I wanted them to take our product and feel better in the shortest time possible.

I wanted another liquid product, and I wanted it to taste good so that patients could drink it with ease.

Initially, I came up with a total of fourteen whole foods in the formula, with four of the fourteen as the main whole foods to help with pain, inflammation, and arthritis. Because this formula had such great anti-inflammatory properties, and because we chiropractors see tons of patients with inflammation in various areas, I decided to name it Chiropractor's Choice.

Before my team and I released Chiropractor's Choice to the public in 2008, I tested it on my dad. Incredibly, the swelling that he had in his feet for two and a half years started to go away, and he almost instantly started feeling much better. Unfortunately, several of the ingredients in Chiropractor's Choice are non-soluble, which meant that no matter how we tried, the liquid formulation would always taste too gritty for mass consumption. So, in July 2011, we converted Chiropractor's Choice to capsule form. We took our best ingredients from the original formula and put them in a capsule. They are sea cucumber, stabilized rice bran, *Boswellia serrata,* sea kelp, and milk thistle. The feedback has been tremendously positive.

Sea Cucumber

I believe that this whole food is the best joint supplement on the planet for humans mainly because our family trees are linked. Ancestors of sea cucumbers (more than 540 million years ago) gave rise to the super phylum of animals that included chordates (humans) and echinoderms (sea cucumbers). Modern research has been linked to sea cucumbers being beneficial for normal structure in musculoskeletal inflammatory diseases, especially rheumatoid arthritis, osteoarthritis, and ankylosing spondylitis, a rheumatic disease that affects the spine.

Stabilized Rice Bran

We use a form of stabilized rice bran that contains more than 110 known antioxidants along with high quantities of water-soluble vitamins, particularly B complex. Our supplier has licenses for many patents that include formulations for treating inflammatory diseases.

Boswellia serrata

Boswellia serrata, also known as frankincense, is a gum resin extracted from the bark of a tree in India. It contains boswellic acids that allay inflammation by stopping or slowing down the body's pro-inflammatory mediators such as leukotrienes. *Boswellia serrata* has been clinically studied and proven to have positive effects on many inflammatory diseases, from arthritis to asthma to Crohn's disease.

Sea Kelp

Sea kelp contains organic sources of various nutrients, including vitamins, trace minerals, minerals, amino acids, antioxidants, and much more. As mentioned, sea-based nutrition thrives in a salt-water based environment, which is similar to the makeup of 70–80 percent of the human body. Sea kelp is neither plant nor animal but classified in a group known as algae. The sea kelp that we use in this formula is *Ascophyllum nodosum*, and it is one of the sea vegetables present in the SeaAloe formula. Again, over 2000 studies have been conducted on sea vegetation and how sea vegetables help to normalize cellular health. They are perfectly suited for our biology.

Milk Thistle (Silymarin)

Many professional herbalists recommend milk thistle extract to support normal response to various inflammatory conditions as well as liver disorders, including viral hepatitis, fatty liver (associated with long term alcohol use), and liver damage from drugs and industrial toxins such as carbon tetrachloride.

Additional Fuels

In addition to liquid fuel, probiotics and DHA (an omega-3 fatty acid called docosahexaenoic acid) should be included in a daily regimen. They are invaluable additions to a healthy lifestyle.

Probiotics

It's important to take a probiotic 10–30 minutes after breakfast and/or dinner each day. Probiotics help to replenish valuable **good bacteria** present in the colon. Maintaining normal amounts of these **good bacteria** helps maintain the delicate microbial balance in our bodies. Probiotics play an important role in promoting a healthy digestive process and immune function.

Throughout our daily lives, the quantity of good bacteria in our bodies diminishes as a result of stress, poor diet, antibiotics, and antibacterial wipes and cleaners. We actually ingest less good bacteria each day than we should. This is why it is absolutely paramount to take a good, daily probiotic. According to Dr. D'Adamo's GenoType research, eating the right probiotic for your blood type is also essential because beneficial bacteria use our blood as their food supply—so it's best to ingest the probotics that respond positively to our individual blood types. {See appendix for my recommendations.}

Furthermore, *Lactobacillus* strains of bacteria synthesize many of the essential B, A, and K vitamins in the gut that are available to the host. If you cannot afford a probiotic, then simply buy a purely natural yogurt. Make sure that the labels do not read low sugar, no sugar added, or less sugar. If you see *low sugar* or *less sugar* written on the label, be aware that it will more than likely contain artificial sugars. This is a clever marketing strategy by product manufacturers. Yogurt won't fully replenish all the good bacteria in your colon, but it will certainly help.

Quick Reference: *What can probiotics do for me?*

- Beneficial effects on intestinal microbial balance
- Prevention of intestinal tract infection
- Reduction of lactose intolerance
- Reduction of inflammatory and allergic reactions
- Regulation of gut motility
- Beneficial effect on urogenital and *H. pylori* infections

DHA

DHA is the most abundant **omega-3 fatty acid** in the human body especially when we are talking about the nervous system. DHA is the number one brain food...period. In fact, look at some of the following facts about DHA:

- Accounts for 97 percent of the omega-3 fats in the brain
- Accounts for 93 percent of the omega-3 fats in the retina
- Key component in heart tissue
- Naturally found in breast milk

Many scientific studies have proven that DHA has positive health benefits for everyone from pregnant or nursing mothers and infants, to healthy adults and the elderly. Increased levels of DHA have also been **shown to improve** cholesterol, decrease the risk of eye disorders like age-related macular degeneration (ARMD), glaucoma, and dry eye syndrome (DES), and lower the risk of cognitive disorders like Alzheimer's disease and dementia. DHA can be found in various infant formulas, organic milk, and egg products. Look specifically for DHA on products you buy at your grocery store.

I believe we should take DHA from algae daily. Don't use fish or fish oil. Fish get their DHA from somewhere—and that somewhere is algae. Why not go to the source? {See appendix for my recommendations.}

Quick Reference: *What can DHA do for me?*

- Brain and central nervous system development and function
- Psychomotor development (such as hand-eye coordination)
- Visual development and function
- Heart health
- Nerve signal transmission

A Lifestyle of Awareness

Keeping your body fueled every day of your life is the key to staying younger and more vibrant longer. We are surrounded by foods that aren't nutritious or healthy for us. We're constantly tempted to eat processed, GMO-foods. It's impossible not to eat them, really. What *is* possible is to fuel your body with an additive every day. Here's my routine:

I wake up in the morning and immediately drink 20 ounces of water along with three algae-based DHA softgels. For adults, I recommend 600–800 milligrams of DHA per day.

When I've finished my water, I take Superfruits GT, after which I eat breakfast and drink a cup of coffee.

At the end of the day, after dinner, I take SeaAloe and a probiotic, which is particularly helpful with digestive issues.

At the very minimum, taking Superfruits GT in the morning and SeaAloe in the evening provides the body with twenty-three different whole foods that you can't get in your normal diet! Fast forward fifteen or twenty years of consistent fuel that matches what your body really thrives on: your engine will run better than the average person your age because you have consistently and daily applied this fuel additive.

The most difficult part of this process for most people is discipline. It's easy to rush out of the house without your morning dose, or to doze off on the couch at night and skip your evening regimen. But let me reiterate that you are in this for the long haul. You are walking around with this amazing machine *that needs the right fuel*.

Then, believe it or not, there are ways to enhance your health to an even higher level, once you have your fuel routine established. These include understanding your nervous system better, pinpointing what factors are affecting your nervous system, and making sure to repair your nervous system when it breaks down. I call this the lifestyle of awareness, which includes watching and listening to the signs our bodies communicate to us.

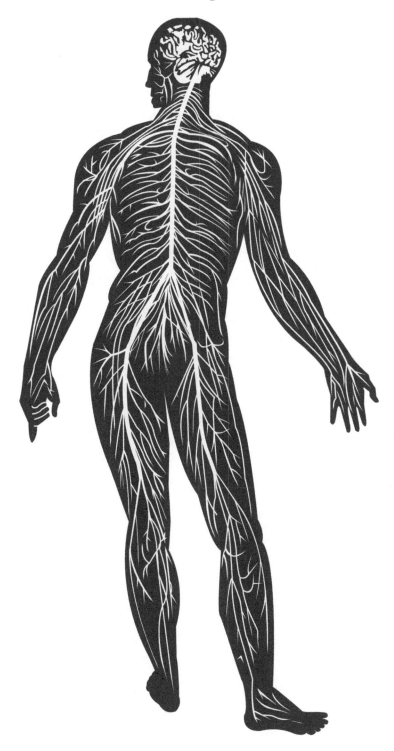

PART II

Maintaining the
Brain-to-Body
Connection

TESTIMONIAL: *MISSY CORMIER*

Two of our children, Hayden and Molly, were afflicted with Molluscum contagiosum, which is a pox virus and looks like a bunch of small warts all over the skin. It's extremely contagious and very common. Our daughter started getting the molluscum that her older brother had endured for years right around the time my husband, Chris, started researching ways to expand and energize his chiropractic practice using supplements, nerve health, brain-body connectivity, and Quantum Neurology®.

We had both been frustrated with traditional medicine since Hayden's birth. He had been sick so much. He'd contracted a MRSA staph infection; his tonsils had to be removed; he, like me, suffered terrible allergies. Chris was determined to find a better way to keep his family healthy.

I was threatened and scared by what seemed to me like hocus pocus—this wasn't traditional medicine, or even traditional chiropractic. I didn't want Chris to put himself in a vulnerable position. I didn't want him to get into trouble doing anything out there. What I had to remember was that nothing Chris ever does will do more damage than what people are doing to themselves already.

He definitely wanted to explore helping people in a more efficient manner. He kept telling me stories to try and convince me of the efficacy of Quantum Neurology®, but I didn't want to hear it.

One day, when Molly's molluscum had spread all over her body, Chris treated her with a Quantum Neurology® technique. Within two days, hundreds of molluscum on my child's body had vanished. I went to give her a bath, and I ran my hand up her arm, and it was smooth. I looked at Chris and I said, "What did you do to her?" and he said, "That's this new technique. Missy, Quantum Neurology® works." Chris explained that Quantum Neurology® made Molly's brain recognize the virus faster and, therefore, fight it faster on its own.

When I saw it with my own eyes, I truly understood what Chris meant when he kept saying that the body can heal itself. If

I had not witnessed it in my own child, I would've been skeptical forever.

I let my guard down a bit, and gave Chris my blessing. Ever since then, our kids have been so much healthier than they were when they first started out. I, too, am healthier at 37 than I was at 22. I don't know how that's possible except to say that I have a better connection between my brain and my body. There's nothing interrupting it anymore. The last antibiotic I took was four and a half years ago, which is saying something for a person who was on antibiotics every month for many years.
--Missy Cormier

Chapter 3: *Understanding Our Connections*

The Breaker Box Brain

If you have ever said to yourself something like "it's all in my head" when you feel terrible, you are right. It *is* all in your head. Your brain's level of functionality determines how you feel every day. Everything involving your health exists in your brain. We live in a world with a broad range of individual neurological functions.

From the professional athlete to the arthritic 90-year-old great-grandmother, the brain's neurological connections to the body vary from person to person on a spectrum of neurological health. Everyone's different. In general, we rely on doctors and health professionals to outline the proper path to health for us. Unfortunately, most times the instructions are not tailored to our individual bodies or, worse, are just plain guesswork. Long-term maintenance requires more than a ballpark estimate as a treatment plan. Now more than ever, I want people to understand their *own* bodies and how to repair them so that they can make informed decisions concerning health.

When my father became ill, I was forced to think outside the box to find a solution for him. Traditional medicine wasn't phasing his ailments. Traditional chiropractic wasn't doing anything for him either. It's funny how looking at the world from a new angle changes your perspective on everything. As a result, I have a way of looking at the human body that situates optimum health precisely in brain connectivity and repairs the broken connections through a series of techniques that underlie Quantum Neurology® (see Chapter 4).

I began seeing the brain as a complex breaker box; while the average number of breaker switches in your house is thirty, your brain houses thousands of breakers, and, while all brains are anatomically the same, we tend to forget that each brain, like each fingerprint, is unique—particularly in how it reacts to stimulus. Depending on your genetics and lifestyle, your brain might actually *like* certain things that other brains don't.

This isn't something we usually hear, but your brain's likes and dislikes will actually influence how many breakers are "on" and how many are "off" between your brain and your body. You might have one hundred breakers off, your neighbor, only twenty-five…your best friend, just ten.

The way you feel right now is a representation of which breakers are on and which breakers are off in your brain. When you experience symptoms like pain or numbness, your pain is actually signaling a tripped breaker situation. Simply put, if your leg has been throbbing in the same spot for weeks, some breakers that connect your leg to your brain have been switched off.

In essence, every disease on earth has the same general diagnosis: tripped breakers in the brain. The most important component to feeling good every day, and to becoming less vulnerable to illness, is your brain's connectivity to these four parts:

ORGANS	BONES
MUSCLES	SKIN

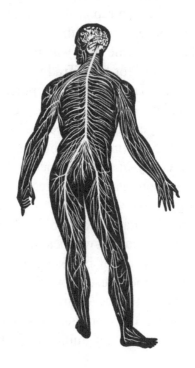

Organs

All of your organs—your heart, lungs, gallbladder, digestive tract, kidneys, liver and so on—have individual nerve connections to the brain. Groups of organs make up various systems of your body: musculoskeletal, cardiovascular, digestive, endocrine, integumentary, urinary, lymphatic, immune, respiratory, reproductive, and last—but really first—the incredible nervous system.

- The cardiovascular system is comprised primarily of the heart, arteries, veins, and capillaries. The digestive system consists of the parotid glands, salivary glands, esophagus, stomach, small intestine, large intestine.
- The integumentary system is the largest organ system because it has all the skin as well as sweat and sebaceous glands, hair, nails, and arrectores pilorum (small muscles at the root of each hair which contract to cause goose bumps).
- The lymphatic system is comprised of the spleen, lymph nodes, and vessels spread throughout the entire body.
- The respiratory system is comprised primarily of the lungs, bronchi, and trachea.
- The musculoskeletal system consists of all the bones, joints, muscles, tendons, and ligaments. As a side note, the typical adult human has approximately 206 bones and approximately 640 skeletal muscles within the body.
- The urinary system is comprised of the kidneys, bladder, ureters, and urethra.
- The reproductive system is comprised of different groups of organs in men (primarily the testes, prostate, and penis) and women (primarily the ovaries, uterus, and vagina).
- The endocrine system is where your metabolism and hormones are derived. Faults in the organs of

this system lead to major problems like diabetes and obesity. Organs within this system are the pituitary, hypothalamus, pineal, thyroid, parathyroid, thymus, adrenals, gonads, pancreas, and so on, with slight variations in hierarchy from male to female.

In order for peak body function to occur, every single one of the aforementioned organs in the various systems needs to be connected by wires from the brain in order to properly communicate. This is where the nervous system comes into play as a massive system of millions of human wires called nerves that connect to your brain via the spinal cord and brain stem. When a hormone is secreted properly by the thyroid, for instance, it's because your brain has a good connection to its thyroid.

My wife has a prevalent history of cancer in her family. Both of her parents and her two sisters have had thyroid cancer. Before I developed the repair system, one lobe of my wife's thyroid swelled to the size of a baseball. She had an ultrasound, which showed a plethora of cysts in that lobe. Then she had a biopsy, which indicated precancerous cells. So, her doctors naturally wanted to remove that section of the thyroid.

Looking back on all this now, I realize that a thyroid would never grow cysts under normal circumstances—when your brain is properly connected to your thyroid. On the flip side, when your brain is not connected to your thyroid for a long enough period of time, events like cysts can occur. We should be more concerned about restoring the connectivity before this sort of reaction even occurs.

My wife had half of her thyroid removed. Thankfully, the surgeon was able to keep the other half of her thyroid in place. Since that time, and as I've been developing the repair system, my wife has been on no thyroid medication. Zero. Her body has maintained normal thyroid hormone levels—even during her last pregnancy. Any doctor she sees is perplexed. The simple fact is that through fueling and repairing my wife's body correctly and keeping her brain more connected to her various parts, she is a healthier person.

The Digestive Tract

Many doctors and nutritional specialists are talking about the digestive tract. That's because there are an estimated 500 million neurons (nerve cells) and nearly a mile of twists and turns in the gastrointestinal tract alone. Some people are actually calling it the second brain. Think about that. How important is the gastrointestinal tract? Every time you swallow something, your body has to know what to do with it, what to use, what to discard. The moment you put something on your tongue, your brain and body begin communicating. We taste salt, sweet, bitter, sour, and umami (a savory, meaty-type taste). There are three different nerves that go to the tongue from the brainstem and give it taste capability. Those nerves are cranial nerves VII (facial), X (vagus), IX (glossopharyngeal). If one of these nerves has a weak signal, every time a certain taste comes into contact with your tongue, breakers in your body start shutting off. Like an alarm system, your whole nervous system gets compromised, and other parts will also begin to shut down. Moving from the mouth down through the esophagus, we find the stomach where stomach acid breaks down food in preparation for the next part of the digestive tract. We all hear a great deal on television commercials about the negative effects of stomach acid, but we actually need the stuff for digestion. Whenever someone has heartburn or gastroesophageal reflux disease, it's because there's a disconnection between the brain and the nerves that go to the upper, or lower gastrointestinal tract, *not* because the body needs over-the-counter acid reducing medicine. If various regions are disconnected, the digestion process doesn't flow as it should.

After the stomach breaks down the food you've swallowed, assuming the stomach works properly with no leaking acid, the food moves to the small intestine, where nutrients are absorbed. Your small intestine knows which nutrients to extrapolate and where to send them. In the various parts of your large intestine, where the food goes next, the remnants of the food are converted into waste. Your body switches from absorption to waste-removal mode. If your brain is connecting properly to the large intestine, waste gets properly assimilated and moves out of your body. All of that tubing must have a good connection to the brain. Without it, your digestive tract won't do its job.

The Gallbladder Dilemma

The gallbladder—where bile is stored after secretion by the liver and before release into the intestines—won't help you properly digest your food without an adequate wiring connection to your brain. The gallbladder doesn't exist in a vacuum. There is a nerve connection between the gallbladder and the brain. This wire is traditionally the L1 nerve, which wraps around from the lumbar spine and runs to the gallbladder. You often hear about people having their gallbladders removed—most often because their gall bladders were either full of gallstones and/or not functioning. A malfunctioning gallbladder makes people feel awful, causing painful indigestion, bloating, back pain, and shoulder pain.

The body sends off major signals when the gallbladder stops working. In my first years of practice, patients would come in with right shoulder pain, and I knew even then that the pain was referred from the gallbladder. I'd send them out for an ultrasound, which would initially come back normal. I could temporarily alleviate symptoms with my old method of spine adjustments as I loosened the musculature in the right places, but the pain would inevitably return with repeated bouts of indigestion and referred pain into the right shoulder. A year later, I'd send the patient for another ultrasound and—lo-and-behold—we'd see some gall stones or some signs of dysfunction in the gallbladder.

The body is made with backups, which means other body parts can fill in for the malfunctioning one, but once you start experiencing extreme signs and symptoms, the wiring has disconnected. A prolonged weak brain to gallbladder connection leads to undue pressure on the liver, parts of the small intestine, parts of the stomach, and the pancreas which collaboratively have to overcompensate. Instead of simply fixing the disconnection, in today's world we wait until that part has failed—and then we decide to yank it out. When I began to reconnect the right wires from the brain to the gallbladder, the symptoms would disappear.

In the Office: *The Pregnancy Miracle*

A young woman came to the office desperate that she couldn't get pregnant, despite *in vitro* fertilization on several occasions. When we met, I reminded her that while I'm not a fertilization specialist I could check her ovary, uterus, and fallopian tube connections to her brain. I did, and the connections were extremely weak, with almost no communication between the brain and these organs. In the female body the pancreas, thymus, parathyroid, and pineal gland will act as backup hormone producers when the ovaries are not well connected. In this patient, though, the pancreas and thyroid were also poorly connected to the brain. Her connections were failing in a domino effect pattern. She had neck pain, which indicated a wiring problem to the parathyroid, and lower back pain, which indicated wiring issues to the ovaries, uterus, and pancreas. We zoned in on these areas in several sessions, and by reconnecting them, the probability that this patient would conceive was heightened. Within two months, she was pregnant.

In the Office: *The $15,000 Bowel Movement*

I recently saw a teenage patient whose parents brought her into the office desperate for a solution to their daughter's mysterious and unrelenting abdominal pain. This patient had been in and out of hospitals for weeks; she'd had blood work, an MRI, a CT scan, a lower gastrointestinal scope, and a HIDA scan (which helps track bile from the liver to the small intestine). Every test came back negative or inconclusive, yet the patient was consistently doubled over in pain despite taking multiple prescribed medications. I spent about fifteen minutes with this patient and pinpointed neurologically where her brain-body disconnection was occurring. For this patient, peristalsis, which is the wavelike contraction that massages food through the gastrointestinal tract from mouth to anus, had slowed in several places. As a result, fecal matter had become severely compacted, causing drastic pain. Her parents didn't need to spend thousands and thousands of dollars—$15,000 to be exact—before finding this out. Using pinpointing techniques, I found her problem and administered a treatment plan in one reasonable office visit. Within two days, this teenager's pain was gone.

Bones

Technically bones are organs, but I give them a separate classification because there are so many (approximately 206), and because they play a vital role in the daily functionality of the body. Bones are our framework and they help to keep us upright as well as protecting vital organs. The average human body produces one trillion blood cells per day. Those one trillion blood cells come primarily from a collaborative effort of all the bones in your body to produce your blood.

Most of your blood gets produced in your bone marrow, so if you have a weak brain-to-bone connection, your blood won't be as healthy as it would be if your bones and your brain were communicating properly. If your brain has a bad connection to your femur, for instance, where the majority of bone marrow gets produced, problems will begin to unfold with respect to the quality of your blood. In turn, your brain-to-blood connection is weaker, and you become more vulnerable to common occurrences like wasp stings. A simple event that your body would normally fight off within minutes can suddenly veer into a dramatic downward spiral, causing infection and swelling all over your body. The traditional medical route is to put a patient on antibiotics and steroids, which actually reduce immunity. But, look at the root of the problem; it's a brain-to-bone connection issue.

In the Office: *Allergic Reaction*

I recently had a patient who came into my office swollen and red from head to toe from a sting. It was the worst case of allergic reaction I've seen. I re-linked this patient's brain-to-bone connection; we made the brain happier with (less allergic to) its own blood. Literally within twenty-four hours, this patient was 100 percent recovered—no swelling, no redness.

This isn't my healing patients; this is helping the body heal itself. What's more, if it's running properly before you get stung, these events can be prevented altogether!

Muscles

Just like bones are organs, technically muscles are also, but, again, I give them a separate classification because there are so many (approximately 640 skeletal muscles and countless smooth muscles in organs and vessels). You can look at any neurology textbook and find an explanation about how every part of your body has a neurological activation that comes from the spinal cord and moves to a particular region. All of your muscles must have nerve connections from the brain, otherwise they don't work. Take the extensor hallucis longus, a muscle that controls the extension of your big toe. The extensor hallucis longus connects to the brain through the L5 nerve root, which is in the lumbar spine. The last lumbar nerve runs on either side of your spinal cord, through your buttock, into your leg, and down into the extensor hallucis longus at the front portion of your tibia. If the connection between your brain and that muscle is weaker than it should be, you're going to have problems lifting your big toe.

In the Office: *Disc Herniation*

My dad is once again a great example because he had issues at an early age with the rigors of farm life and had a massive disc herniation in his lower back, the disc pushing on the L5 nerve root. My dad's foot started dropping when he walked. He couldn't pick up his toes. In his first surgery, at twenty years of age, they took the herniated disc off the L5 nerve. Unfortunately, no one at that time was doing Quantum Neurology® repair techniques, so he went into the surgery with a paralyzed muscle (zero on a scale of zero to five: zero being no movement and five being normal neurological strength). When he recovered from that surgery, he was only at a one or two out of five. The doctor who treated my dad told him that, while his disc was fixed, he would have permanent nerve damage. To the doctor's credit, he recommended exercise and walking for my dad. Once I tested my dad and performed Quantum Neurology® techniques on him years later, his foot went from a two or three after years of exercise to a five…immediately. We took the nerve that had been damaged for 30-plus years, and we turned that nerve back on simply by restoring the brain's connectivity to that muscle. This possible recovery is true for every single muscle in the body.

Skin

The skin, too, is technically an organ, but I give it a separate classification because it is the largest organ in the whole body. Think about this. If I'm going to walk up to something and touch it with my eyes closed, my brain has to know exactly what to do, and fast, to detect if it's hot, cold, sharp, smooth. It has to be able to interpret light and vibration. A wire fires from skin to brain, and then the brain responds to the stimulus. Every inch of your skin must have a nerve connection to your brain. Skin has to sense everything it comes into contact with. As I'm reading this over, one of my hands is sitting on a mouse. If my brain has a good connection with my palm, it will understand what I'm touching and maneuver the mouse appropriately.

In a diabetic with badly damaged peripheral nerves and polyneuropathy, the hand may lose the ability to sense its surroundings. Someone with polyneuropathy might touch a hot surface and not know it for a few seconds. A person with good connectivity would know in less than a millisecond. Obviously, this could cause all kinds of problems, from burns to infected cuts to bruises that don't heal, and worse. Remember my earlier story in Chapter 2 about the doctor I encountered when I was in college, who had diabetes and had been working barefoot in his dirt garden? Because of the diabetes, and even before, his brain's connection to the skin in his feet hadn't been good for a long time. This doctor didn't take care of his cut, and because his brain was already not connected well to skin, gangrene took over. Again, this could have all been prevented by taking care of the brain-skin connection.

In the Office: *The Skin Saver*

I recently treated a teenager with a patterned skin rash that radiated from her shoulder, down her arms, and over her thumb. It was an obvious case of shingles. Because shingles is a virus and viruses infiltrate cells, fooling them into believing that they, too, are viruses, medication is ineffective. Aside from the fact that she felt devastated about her physical appearance, this patient was obviously suffering from weak connections from her brain to the right side of her body. I went in and strengthened those areas, mostly branching from the C6 nerve, and within four treatments, the shingles had disappeared completely.

Human Kryptonite

Statistically speaking, the more you do to prevent neurological dysfunction, the higher the probability that you'll stay healthy! So, how do we avoid tripped breakers to the brain? Well, we can't *always* avoid them without some outside help, as you'll see in Chapter 4, but in addition to keeping every cell in your body strong with fuel, there *are* some triggers—stressors to the human body—we can avoid and specific ways to counteract what I call human kryptonite. As with Superman's glowing green nemesis, these human poisons can interfere with brain-to-body connective health, stressing your body until it begins to break down. By being aware of some universal kryptonite stressors (you'll recognize a few from Chapter 2), you will reduce the chances of your brain-to-body breakers switching off as frequently, or in large numbers. Human kryptonite includes:

- Bad Posture
- Pathogens
- Poor Diet and Nutrition
- Sleep Deprivation
- Laboratory-Made Prescription Drugs
- Laboratory-Made Vitamins
- Environment: Toxins and Elements
- Mental and Emotional Stress

Bad Posture

Think about the position you're holding your body in right now. Are you hunched over this book? Are you curled into a ball in bed? Are you craning your neck? We're constantly squeezing cell phones between our ear and shoulder while cooking dinner; we're hunched over computers; we're leaning over plates of food in front of the TV; we're sitting at too-low computer screens. Our bodies weren't made for these contortions.

We can take care of our bodies by practicing just a few techniques that keep us better aligned on a daily basis:

Practice symmetrical posturing every day by trying to keep your body even on both sides.

The following are the **most common fixes you can** make each day with respect to your posture:

Cell Phone Neck. Talking on one ear consistently causes asymmetry in the body by repeatedly contracting the same group of muscles on one side of your body—the arm is bent at a strange angle, the neck leans to one side. Whenever you're talking on the phone, alternate ears or get a hands-free set or headset.

Butt Wallet Syndrome. When you build a house, you don't make one side of your house higher than the other; if you do, your roof will be crooked. Likewise, if you stick something in your rear pocket, and you sit on it throughout the day, you're heightening the probability that you're going to turn off breakers in your body due to muscular tension. Do not put your wallet or anything else in your rear pockets. Instead, place all things in your front pockets.

Crooked Computer Syndrome. When your computer screen is not situated directly in front of you, you force your neck to perform unnatural acrobatics. If your head is bent down, for instance, you've reduced the normal lordotic curvature in the neck. Do not place your computer screen off to the right or left. Instead, place your computer screen directly in front of you at eye level.

Butt Tuck Syndrome. Slouching compresses the discs in the lumbar spine, which allows for a greater possibility of irritated nerves and disc degeneration, heightening the probability of a herniated disc. Do not slouch all day long while you are sitting, standing, or squatting. Do this instead: Focus on keeping a little arch in your lower back all the time—while sitting, standing, or squatting.

Mouse Disease. If you consistently keep the hand and arm that operates your mouse higher than the opposite hand and arm, that side of your body will be tilted, contracting more musculature, causing more nerve firing in that area of the body. Do not have your computer mouse placed high up where your right shoulder is higher than your left. Instead, place your mouse where you can keep both of your shoulders even and relaxed.

Same Leg Crossing Disease. Do not consistently cross your left leg over your right leg or vice versa. Instead, make sure to alternate sides. Cross the left then the right; that way, you won't be shifting your pelvis continuously on that side, heightening the potential for joint irritation as well as neurological damage.

Stomach Sleeper's Disease. Do not sleep on your stomach. Instead, sleep on your back or on your side, and use a good neck pillow. {See appendix for my recommendations.} Sleeping on your side or back lessens the probability of sleeping asymmetrically. The neck pillow I recommend supports good side and back sleeping.

Do a Jig: *The Vagus Nerve*

The most important nerve in the whole entire body is the vagus nerve. This nerve supplies power to your voice in addition to almost all of your organs. Because this nerve has so many connections to different body parts, it tends to suffer more disconnects than other nerves. An easy way to help improve the connectivity of the vagus nerve to all the parts of the body is something I call the Crazy Exercise. Simply, the exercise involves walking or jogging in place while talking and moving your arms. Make sure to move your arms and legs while reciting the alphabet or singing your favorite song. I nicknamed it the Crazy Exercise because, well, it seems crazy when somebody tells you to talk to yourself and jump around—but if you look at cardiovascular studies, talking and walking has been proven to increase your endurance. My understanding of this phenomenon is on the neurological level, though. You *could* walk and talk with a partner, but that requires more planning. By performing the Crazy Exercise at various intervals during the day for a few minutes at a time, you're turning on the brain's connection to lots of different muscles. Talking turns on the vagus nerve, or cranial nerve X. All the cranial nerves are in back of your brain stem, and one of those nerves, X, the vagus nerve, is the most important nerve in the entire body because it literally goes to almost every organ and provides energy to almost every part of the body. As you're walking and/or jumping around, you're stimulating your brain's connection to your musculature, and as you begin talking you're turning on your vagus nerve, which stimulates the vagus connection to all your organs.

Pathogens in Our Bodies

In the human body, we're seeing more types of pathogens entering the nervous system and actually turning it off. We have to safeguard people with neurogenic immunity, which means keeping the nervous system intact and aware with respect to all the areas of the brain that connect to the immune system. As you saw in Chapter 2, this is something I feel really strongly about. We are literally forcing pathogens to evolve at the fastest pace in history—through our own actions. Our bodies have to keep up with this, have to understand what's good and bad— and they can if treated properly. Right now, there are only 100,000 named species of fungi, but there's an estimated 1.5 million species of fungi actually living in the world today, which means there's a minimum of 1.4 million fungi with no name![3] We have to strengthen our nervous systems with respect to these pathogens—especially children. My youngest son is two, and I have a five-year-old daughter and an eight-year-old son, and they're encountering exponentially more pathogens than previous generations ever did. That said, you can't stay away from these things. I'm not writing this book to foster paranoia. I'm banking on the fact that awareness is half the battle. Nerve health in the form of fuel and repair is the key to solving the pathogen problem.

Like it or not, bad pathogens are in your body right now. They get into your sinuses, mouth, ears, bladder, nose, eyes, and other areas. Examples of how this happens are fungal spores brought into your lungs from the air that your breathe, viruses and bacteria brought into your body by rubbing your eyes, or parasites brought into your body from a particular food. These pathogens are constantly looking for a place to settle down.

So, if you already have a weak brain connection to a part of your body, an opportunistic pathogen can invade and attack, forming a small colony inside of you. The brain will

---

[3]Hawksworth DL. (2006). "The fungal dimension of biodiversity: magnitude, significance, and conservation". *Mycological Research* **95** (6): 641–655. doi:10.1016/S0953-7562(09)80810-1.

think this new pathogen is a friend because the pathogen has entered a weakened neurological area of the body, and the body is incapable of a normal search-and-destroy reaction for an invading pathogen. Next thing you know, you have dozens of supposed "friends" living at your house, spending all of your money, eating all of your food while you are working hard every day. You go home each night exhausted from a hard day's work; you have no food or money because your "friends" have used them up. You wake up exhausted and start all over again.

First, you need to protect yourself as much as possible with the right fuels. Second, you need someone to come into your system and un-brainwash it by telling it to kill off all of these supposed "friends" so that they will stop sucking the life out of you. This is where repairs and updates to your neurological system have become an absolute necessity. In Chapter 4, you'll learn more about how to train your brain to fight off these bad pathogens so that your immune system develops memory and keeps up with fast evolving and morphing pathogens. Washing your hands before touching your eyes, ears, nose, or mouth might be one of the easiest ways to protect yourself each day.

Nutrition and Diet: *What Not to Consume*

Nutrition and diet are an almost impossibly large category. There are so many artificial ingredients and processed foods in our diets. As you've seen, a good whole food supplement can provide many of the good nutrients we're missing from our diets, but in order to live a truly healthy life, there are certain additives to avoid religiously.

Avoid artificial sugars, especially aspartame, sucralose, phenylalanine, saccharin (e.g., NutraSweet*, Equal*, Splenda[4*]), chewing gum except all-natural {See appendix for my recommendation}, diet drinks and sodas, low sugar and sugar-free products.

If you're thinking that this list pretty much eliminates the possibility of eating sweets, you're wrong. You can use organic sugar in moderation, or if you want to use products with lower sugar and lower glycemic indexes, then use stevia, luo han guo, or agave nectar products.

Despite what most people believe, your several trillion cells need sugar to function properly each day. If you look at the body on a chemical level, 99.5 percent of the body is comprised of twelve of the 118 elements. The top three elements present are oxygen, carbon, and hydrogen. The chemical formula for sugar consists of small amounts of carbon, hydrogen, and oxygen; our bodies need sugar. Sugar has never been the problem in the body—just excessive amounts of it. At one point, we had this opportunity in our country to start limiting the amount of sugar in products. As processed food started becoming the norm, our country's leaders could have taken a stand by passing laws to limit grams of sugar per serving in processed foods. Why is it necessary for soft drinks to have thirty grams of sugar? Instead of mandating that the food companies not put so much sugar in their products, we got the bright idea to start using sugar substitutes.

[4*] *The use of NutraSweet®, Equal®, and Splenda®, are logos, trademarks, or registered trademarks of their respective owners. Use of these logos, trademarks, or registered trademarks is for reference only and does not imply any connection or relationship between this book and these products.*

Take aspartame as a case in point. In 1965, a scientist named James M. Schlatter discovered aspartame by accident. He was doing a lab experiment for an anti-ulcer drug. He licked his finger after doing the experiment and tasted this incredibly sweet stuff...lo and behold *that's how we have aspartame-filled products.*

Artificial sugars, collaboratively, are much sweeter than natural sugar. Real sugar comes from naturally grown sugar cane, but where does artificial sugar come from? A laboratory filled with chemicals. Did you know that aspartame, when heated to 98.6 degrees (your normal body temperature), breaks down chemically into several dangerous substances, including formaldehyde—the chemical used to stiffen and preserve human cadavers.

Even if we eliminate the fact that artificial sugars are bad for you, you're still ingesting something much sweeter than sugar, 150 or more times sweeter, and your taste buds become acclimated to that particular taste. What does that mean to you when you eat regular sugar? You're going to want more. Not to mention, people who eat lots of artificial sugars have unhealthy nervous systems. So use common sense. Don't avoid eating sugar. Simply eat sugar in moderation and avoid excessive amounts in one sitting.

If you do happen to ingest three or more simple carbohydrates, which act like pure sugar in your system, or if you are worried about eating real sugar and controlling your blood sugar levels, then do the following immediately after consuming sugar products: walk around the block, do ten standing squats, ten push-ups, ten pull-ups, ten walking lunges. Exercising immediately after ingesting sugar is a free way to control your own blood sugar levels. Or do the Crazy Exercise!

Avoid eating all foods and seasonings containing MSG (monosodium glutamate). MSG is a flavor enhancer commonly added to Chinese food, canned vegetables, soups, and processed meats, as well as many seasoning mixes. MSG is to salt what artificial sweeteners are to sugar. The more salt your body gets, the more it wants. MSG has been used as a food additive for decades. Here in Louisiana, we have a lot of local people making seasoning blends full of MSG. Over the years, the FDA has received many reports of adverse reactions to foods containing MSG, and I've seen it firsthand. These reactions are known as MSG Symptom Complex and include the following symptoms:

- Headache
- Flushing
- Sweating
- Facial pressure or tightness
- Numbness, tingling, or burning in face, neck, and other areas
- Rapid, fluttering heartbeats (heart palpitations)
- Chest pain
- Nausea
- Weakness

While symptoms are usually mild and generally limited to thirstiness and bloating, why would you do that to your body? By staying away from MSG, you're keeping your body from having to work too hard to digest your food.

In addition to avoiding these things, seeking care from a healthcare professional specializing in the SWAMI GenoType Diet software formulated by Dr. Peter D'Adamo is essential. Dr. D'Adamo has created this software modeled after his GenoType Diet. A group of healthcare professionals in the U.S. have purchased Dr. D'Adamo's computerized methodology to decipher the proper foods for individual patients. This revolutionary software tests blood, saliva, fingerprints, body measurements, teeth characteristics, and much more. In my office, we utilize these test results to assign personalized GenoType Diets ™ with a thirty to forty page report of dietary recommendations consisting of lists of foods that enhance your GenoType and foods to limit or avoid, in addition to meal plans and recipes. Eating the right foods for your personalized GenoType is a surefire way to help your body's chemistry stay in balance, decreasing the likelihood of neurological dysfunction.

Sleep Deprivation

Your pineal gland, a tiny gland behind your eyes, produces melatonin, which causes you to sleep. If your brain isn't well connected to your pineal gland or eyes, or the parts of your body essential for the sleep process, your sleep will be affected. Emotional scarring or high stress can also alter sleep. As soon as you close your eyes, your brain can start firing about something that's worrying you, and you won't sleep. So, your brain needs to be strengthened against this. Instead of buying synthetic melatonin in your pharmacy or health food store, simply turn on your body's melatonin production yourself.

Sleep in the dark. You can turn on your body's melatonin production by sleeping in total darkness. Turn off all nightlights, lamps, TVs, and so on. Your body is designed similarly to a computer, and it needs down time. This means good sleep.

Distract yourself. If you are having trouble sleeping because you are stressed about something, then you should do something before bedtime that you enjoy in order to stop your conscious mind from thinking about it. This could be playing the Wii ™, watching a movie or a comedian, doing some push-ups, praying, meditating, or reading an enjoyable book. In Chapter 4, I'll talk about more advanced methods to help you sleep.

Laboratory-Made Vitamins

For my entire life, I have been surrounded by the great tasting (but hardly nutritious) Cajun diets of Southern Louisiana. Foods like Cajun boudin (sausage made of pork without the blood, pork liver, heart meat, and rice dressing stuffed into pork casings), fried foods like fried shrimp, Cajun fried turkey, various crawfish recipes, and gumbo (stew or soup consisting primarily of a strong stock, meat or shellfish, a thickener, and the vegetable "holy trinity" of celery, bell peppers, and onion) grace our tables. Everyone knows that Cajun food is really great, but most great Cajun food recipes do not include enough raw fruits or vegetables. As a result, many people in the Cajun Heartland enjoy delicious tasting meals with very little health benefit. If we're going to eat like that, we have to use supplements to get the nutrients we need, but vitamins aren't the answer. As I said in Chapter 2, over the three-or-four-year course of recommending laboratory made vitamins and pills, I made the following observations:

There were side effects from multivitamins, vitamins and supplements, like nausea and skin blushing and flushing, or dark yellow-colored urine. Dark yellow urine means that you are getting too-high dosages vitamins. Because the body gets rid of what it can't process, this is an easy way to visualize the money you're wasting on vitamins.

I personally saw thousands of "undigested pills" on x-rays within the digestive tracts of thousands of my patients.

The bottom line was that there seemed to be little health value in these products for my patients, and as a result, I had an epiphany. I started to flush away all my previous understanding about laboratory-made vitamins and supplements. I returned to the old adage about the simplest answer generally being the best. My epiphany, as you've seen, was that we need to get back to the basics. As I already mentioned in Chapter 2, if the label on your supplement lists vitamins and elements (vitamins A, B, C, D, E, calcium, or magnesium) rather than actual grown whole foods (apples, peaches, pears, asparagus), then it is not natural…period. We need to use the best naturally grown whole foods to give our bodies the highest level of nutrients, and in the proper proportions, each and every day. Nowadays, we can actually do so.

Prescription Drugs:
Pills, Powders, and Potions

A statement from a July 1998 issue of *The American Journal of Medicine* states the following:

> Conservative calculations estimate that approximately 107,000 patients are hospitalized annually for nonsteroidal anti-inflammatory drug (NSAID)-related gastrointestinal (GI) complications and at least 16,500 NSAID related deaths occur each year among arthritis patients alone. The figures of all NSAID users would be overwhelming, yet the scope of this problem is generally under-appreciated.

Again, a year later (June 1999) in the *New England Journal of Medicine* there is a similar statement:

> It has been estimated conservatively that 16,500 NSAID-related deaths occur among patients with rheumatoid arthritis or osteoarthritis every year in the United States. This figure is similar to the number of deaths from the acquired immunodeficiency syndrome and considerably greater than the number of deaths from multiple myeloma, asthma, cervical cancer, or Hodgkin's disease. If deaths from gastrointestinal toxic effects from NSAIDs were tabulated separately in the National Vital Statistics reports, these effects would constitute the 15th most common cause of death in the United States. Yet these toxic effects remain mainly a "silent epidemic," with many physicians and most patients unaware of the magnitude of the problem. Furthermore the mortality statistics do not include deaths ascribed to the use of over-the-counter NSAIDS.

These journal articles are shocking. Over 100,000 people are hospitalized for gastrointestinal (GI) bleeding due to prescribed NSAIDs [Celebrex, Motrin, Feldene, Mobiflex, Ponstel, Bextra (off market), Vioxx (off market), ketoprofen, naproxen (Anaprox), piroxicam (Feldene), sulindac (Clinoril), etc.]. Of those hospitalized, 16,500 die every year, and these values are considered "conservative." More importantly, these figures only include prescription NSAIDs used to treat arthritis and are only in the United States. If prescription and over-the-counter NSAID-related hospitalizations and death rates were counted for not only arthritis, but for all conditions, and throughout the world, the figures would undoubtedly be enormous. If you take those figures and apply them over the many years that this class of drug has been available (since the early 1970s), the numbers would be horrific. Yet, no study to date has attempted to quantify these figures.

Americans take more prescription drugs than any other nationality; conventional and alternative medicine alike have tried to tap into the power of the human body, most of the time resulting solely in the alleviation of symptoms, creation of side effects, or no results at all. Make no mistake, remarkable health discoveries have been made in conventional medicine, but there has always been too much focus on healing people with synthetic products: pills, powders, potions, and things made in labs.

The pharmaceutical industry has tried thousands of combinations of the earth's elements hoping to find a magical cure, with very few side effects, for a single ailment. It's an impossible task that costs inordinate amounts of money. You simply can't individualize every drug to match every individual's DNA. Your DNA is different from anyone else's in the entire world. This means that your insulin is different from anyone else's. Your amazing body produces your DNA matched hormones, pain killers, anti-inflammatories, blood cells, digestive enzymes, anti-depressants, melatonin and so many others. These are different from anyone else's in the entire world. Modern medicine's focus on creating a synthetic blend of what your body has stopped producing—instead of looking at the problem's production center—is precisely why drugs have so many side effects.

We live in the land of huge class-action lawsuits. You can't watch TV without seeing an ad for a lawsuit against a prescription or over-the-counter drug. Why do you think that is? No matter how much the scientists at these pharmaceutical companies want to help us, they simply can't make products that match each person's DNA. They would have to individualize every single bottle of pills! Even if they were capable of this, it would still not solve the underlying problem. A classic example: someone with adrenal fatigue, which results in low energy and general tiredness and inflammation. In this person's body, the wiring connection between the brain and the adrenal glands is not sound. The traditional treatment is to take an adrenal fatigue supplement (e.g., cortisone) that mimics what your adrenal glands produce. Inevitably, the supplement won't match exactly what your adrenal glands are producing. A much better way to help this person is to improve the *connection* between the brain and adrenal glands and its counterparts, the hypothalamus and pituitary glands. Improvement of these connections results in the improved production of the adrenal glands.

Let's use the car example again. If you have a hole in your tire, a symptom of that hole will be low air in the tire. What if, instead of repairing the hole, you repeatedly fill up your low tire with air? It's just going to keep deflating. That's common sense. Or, if you've got a bad spark plug, a warning sign might be the check engine light. What if, instead of actually repairing the spark plug, you just cut the wire to your check engine light? Symptom-masking drugs do just that.

On the alternative side of healthcare, too, consumers are spending big bucks on so many different "cures"—many of which have no scientific validity. So many of these vitamin companies claim to be "natural" when they're actually made in a lab just like prescription medication. There are also practitioners rubbing your big toe to cure headaches or blowing cigar smoke on your back to relieve back pain or rubbing snake oils for every malady. What about cure-all potions, pills, powders, suction cups, and electrical frequencies? Many people pop in excess of ten or more supplements or vitamin pills a day! Neither conventional nor alternative medicine is looking at the root cause of disease. They are simply grappling with the symptoms. We need a better solution, one that looks at the whole body, one that sees what can go wrong when the body's connections are weak.

Environmental Toxins

The number one way your body gets rid of toxicity is primarily through your lungs when you breathe, but we live in a world in which not many people practice heavy breathing. When you're out running, for example, your body is doing a lot of breathing and you're getting rid of toxins—that's one of the reasons exercise is so good for you. It forces deep breathing. You may also imbibe toxins outside, but your body should be able to take care of that, too. Because most of us don't engage in heavy breathing, I recommend alternative ways to rid our bodies of environmental toxins. I like to recommend as many options as possible—for anyone from the person who doesn't exercise at all to athletes who train hours and hours daily.

We're constantly ingesting chemicals and toxins through our food, water, and air. If you detoxify your body every day, you're reducing your chances of harmful toxin buildup with harmful side effects. You can do any of the following, hopefully in addition to some exercise that makes you breathe deeply, to help your body get rid of trash each day:

Get some sunlight because it is well known that our bodies benefit tremendously from controlled amounts of the sun's rays. Vitamin D production and body detoxification are just a couple of its main benefits. *If you sweat or perspire during your time in the sun, be sure to bring a towel or cloth to wipe excess perspiration off your skin. You can also take a shower or bath immediately following your time in the sun. Toxins are released from your body (detoxification) when you perspire. You need to get these toxins off your skin to prevent damage to it.*

Take a 15–30 minute hot bath with one cup of sea salt. A sea salt bath helps the body suck toxins out through the skin. It's similar to perspiration in its detoxification qualities.

Get a sauna installed in your home and use it several times per week. Again, the perspiration that a sauna enables is one of the best kinds of detox. Get some detox pads and place them on the bottom of your feet each night. Detox pads literally suck toxicity from your body via your feet. This method is definitely not the most effective, but it offers some hope to those who don't partake in any other detoxification practices.

Avoid heating plastic in the microwave, a process that **can produce harmful byproducts.** Instead, heat food in microwave-safe ceramics and glass. Heating food in a conventional oven or stovetop is much better for you than in microwaves.

Avoid drinking tap water. **Water is the single most important thing that we need each day to live. Pure H2O is hard to come by these days, and, unfortunately, tap water consists of much more than just H2O.** Use bottled water (FIJI* or Aquafina[5*] water is the best) and use a water filter at home for all tap water. Aquafina is one of the only bottled waters on the market that is pure H2O.

Environment: *Elements*

As I've mentioned, only twelve elements make up 99.5 percent of the human body. They are:

- Oxygen 65 percent
- Carbon 18 percent
- Hydrogen 10 percent
- Nitrogen 3 percent
- Calcium 1.5 percent
- Phosphorus 1.2 percent
- Potassium, Sulfur, Chlorine 0.2 percent
- Sodium, Magnesium, Iron 0.05 percent

There are also trace amounts of copper, cobalt, zinc, iodine, selenium, fluorine, manganese, molybdenum, nickel, chromium, and boron in the body, and these elements are necessary for good health. The effects of the elements on the nervous system are a problem I'm working on with Dr. Jim Sheen, a fellow chiropractic physician and Quantum Neurologist, in Nebraska.

[5*]*The use of FIJI® and Aquafina® are logos, trademarks, or registered trademarks of their respective owners. Use of these logos, trademarks, or registered trademarks is for reference only and does not imply any connection or relationship between this book and these products.*

Remember when we began the discussion about your brain's likes and dislikes? When you continuously feed your brain with processed foods, vitamins and supplements saturated with one or more of these elements, you run the risk of the brain rebelling against the excess of that element, or becoming addicted or allergic to said element. This could lead to problems if your brain starts rejecting a vital nutrient. Consistent consumption of anything high in sodium, potassium, or calcium each day will likely cause your brain to become sensitive to sodium, potassium, and/or calcium. Because your body needs sodium, potassium, and calcium for every single neuromuscular contraction to occur, the brain's rejection of these elements becomes dangerous. An example of this that I see routinely is in Restless Leg Syndrome where people experience terrible cramping in the legs at night. This is almost always the result of the body becoming allergic to potassium, which makes inflammation and cramping occur. I have helped countless people get rid of this potassium problem and miraculously the body heals itself by stopping Restless Leg Syndrome.

Brain Addictions

Let's take a closer look at calcium. America is experiencing a calcium-consuming epidemic. Our brains don't know what to do with the countless calcium pills we swallow daily and weird things start happening in the body. For instance:

- Calcium gets deposited in blood vessels, organs, tissues, joints, and ligaments.
- Bones can actually become weaker.
- Energy goes down, and fatigue occurs easily.
- Metabolism slows.
- Muscles experience inconsistent cramping, weakness, or spasms.
- Calcium levels in blood might be high or low.

In addition to supplements, processed foods contain high levels of calcium, too. All of the common wisdom says we need extra calcium, but we don't. We can get appropriate levels of calcium in the foods we eat.

Another example is aluminum, which is not an element present in your body's chemistry. Unfortunately, our bodies come into contact with aluminum very often in our daily routines. Aluminum is commonly found in deodorant, baking powder, and in many pots used for cooking. It isn't a far-fetched hypothesis, and we've all heard it before, that if you routinely ingest and absorb aluminum into your body every day that one day your brain can become sensitive to that element. You don't need aluminum in your body, so your brain should naturally know how to get rid of aluminum if it comes into contact with it. What happens if your brain forgets how to get rid of aluminum because you have a nerve-connection issue?

When the body is inundated with a particular element, a part of the body can actually become a storage site for that unneeded element. If your body develops a weak neurological connection to the pancreas, and you continuously expose yourself to aluminum via deodorant, cooking pots, or aluminum cans, your body may, in time, decide that it doesn't know what to do with aluminum any more. It may begin storing that excess aluminum in the pancreas, a process that makes the brain-body connection even weaker. The chemical makeup of the pancreas does not include aluminum, so if your body is suddenly holding on to it, the brain gets confused and all the pancreas functions—producing digestive enzymes and insulin—become inefficient. Storage of bad elements can happen in any part of the human body.

In the Office: *Blood Sugar Blues*

A patient in his late 40s recently came to my office with low energy; he couldn't perform the normal day-to-day tasks he always had. One day he felt so tired and out of sorts that he drove to the ER to get checked. His blood sugar level was a whopping 840! To put that number into perspective, normal blood sugar is 80–120. The ER doctor—assuming this patient was already diabetic—scolded him for not taking his insulin pills, but this patient had never been diagnosed with diabetes. Needless to say, the patient was put on 72 units of insulin per day, and his blood sugar dropped down to an average of 180 a day, which is better but still too high. His condition resulted in the loss of his treasured pilot's license.

He lived this way, as a 49-year-old diabetic, until he heard about my techniques, so he came to my office. The first thing I told him was that I'm not an endocrinologist or a medical doctor; I'm a chiropractor specializing in the neuromusculoskeletal system but that I would examine him because of his history of neck, middle back, and lower back pain. We checked out his wiring connections. The same wiring that goes to your Sartorius muscle, the L3 nerve, also goes to the pancreas. From the start, this patient had a terrible brain-to-pancreas connection.

Over the course of a few sessions, I began repairing this patient's connectivity, but the connection between the brain and the pancreas was consistently turning off after I turned it on. We came to discover he'd been around aluminum in the course of his career more than any other patient I've ever seen, as a machinist who builds submarine parts. There was aluminum in the pancreas that his body couldn't get rid of. So, *we taught his brain how to get rid of aluminum.* I couldn't consult this patient on his diabetes medications, but I told him that once I started repairing his brain-to-pancreas connections, he would need to monitor his intake with his medical doctor. When the pancreas is functioning properly, it produces insulin and too much administered insulin could result in problems. Within a three-week period this patient was totally off insulin. Within only two months of treatment, he had regained his treasured pilot's license, dusted off his airplane, and begun to fly again. For over a year now, he's been on no diabetic medication whatsoever, and his sugars are always in the normal range.

We can also look at the elements from the angle of the conditions themselves. Let's look at osteoarthritis. At the onset of arthritis, bone spurs, or osteophytes, can grow when calcium accumulates in a particular bone or joint. The body is holding on to, *addicted to*, calcium; it can't remember how to get rid of calcium in that area. We need to teach it how to eliminate calcium in that particular region. So, let's just say, for instance, that the osteoarthritis occurs in the cervical spine—vertebrae C5, C6, and C7, where whiplash occurs. Where the bones and joints start degenerating and calcific deposits start growing on the bones, the spurs work to fuse themselves together. If we educate that person's specific neurology, teaching the brain to give it up, we can teach the body to heal itself.

Brain Allergies

The body can also have an *allergic type* response to a particular element. Let's say a patient has an allergic response to sulfur. Because the ligaments and tendons are made up primarily of sulfates, the body needs sulfur for tendon and ligament maintenance. Let's say you have a rotator cuff injury and have partially torn some tendons. Normally, the body can heal minor tears, but if you've become allergic to sulfur, maybe by ingesting too much of it through food or supplements, you won't heal the same way.

Dr. James Sheen, a fellow Quantum Neurologist in Nebraska, and I have uncovered how to look at the body's chemistry and decipher whether it's addicted or allergic to a certain element through a series of external nerve tests. Remember, if your body is addicted, your brain won't know how to get rid of it. If it's allergic, the brain will forget how to use it and each time it encounters an allergic element, inflammation occurs.

Mental Stress

We're human. We experience the world in both its beauty and its sadness. Deaths, abuse, accidents, traumas, natural disaster, divorce, bad business dealings, illnesses— all have an effect not just on our emotions but on our bodies. So much of our lives are based around the people we love. If that's taken away, because of a death or a break-up, an emotional scar in the brain gets formed. Take divorce, for instance. More than 51 percent of marriages end in divorce, and it's a traumatic event. You begin your marriage by believing the person you're marrying will be your partner forever. All the images of this person with whom you've shared your life, maybe had children with, are stored in your brain. If your marriage ends in divorce, there's a serious emotional scar that has to be dealt with. Otherwise, you might look at your children and be reminded of the negativity of your divorce. This emotional stress can actually translate to physical stress, if allowed. Memories and patterns in your past can interfere with your brain-to-body connectivity.

In the Office: *A Mother's Worry*

I have a patient in her 60s, who is physically very weak, and she's got multiple areas where the nerves aren't connecting. I regularly find these areas and strengthen them, but she's a tough case. She keeps coming back in with weakness in the areas I've strengthened. I looked at factors in her environment: food, drinks, elements in the air, allergies, to no avail. I soon realized, though, that this patient was experiencing severe emotional distress in dealing with her son's difficult divorce. So, this patient was walking out of my office with her physical body much stronger, but she'd leave my office and her brain would immediately pull out these files stored in it. As the worries resonated in her brain, the physical nerves that we turned back on shut off again. She'd leave the office brain-strong and return brain-weak. It became clear that we had to strengthen the mental and spiritual component of her body. As I've said, thoughts, ideas, and memories will always echo in the brain. Negative thoughts resonate so that we'll look for solutions to our future problems, but through brain-body connectivity, we can actually strengthen the brain to deal with these negative thoughts and emotions, giving your brain a little boost in dealing with them.

The human body is simultaneously incredibly complex and beautifully simple. While your brain has complete control over your body all the time, if a particular part of your body loses proper connectivity to your brain for any reason, that body part starts to lose the ability to efficiently do what it normally does. So, while our bodies don't come with instruction manuals, there are road maps that can lead us to optimal health, and these roadmaps include street signs and warnings to stay away from kryptonite. What should you do when vigilance simply isn't enough?

PART III

Quantum Neurology®
Explained

Testimonial: *Desirée Breaux*

I went from having pain everywhere—cramps in my calves, pain in my joints, my neck, my back, my arms—to being virtually pain free after seeing Dr. Cormier. I was able to lose 60 pounds, I think because of the work Dr. C did on my thyroid and parathyroid. My weight gain had probably been from years of eating poorly, but Dr. C allowed me to get into a better place. He works on the connections of the nerves. If I say, "I'm having pain right here where my pancreas is," he says, "Ok, that's the connection to this particular nerve," and he works on that via light therapy and other techniques. One time I was having frequent urination. I had my nieces and nephews with me, and I was basically incontinent. I was mortified. When I went to Dr. Cormier, he pinpointed and adjusted my lower spine with the energy wand, and I haven't had a problem since. Sometimes he uses elements, sometimes he tests to see if I'm allergic to something, but he can always see what's bothering me.

How It Began

When I graduated from chiropractic school, I believed that straightening the spine was the best, most efficient technique in improving the nervous system's functionality. When my loved ones started getting really sick, I realized that what I was doing really wasn't good enough. I had to find more and better ways to strengthen the nervous system.

After releasing Chiropractor's Choice to the public in January of 2008, I started doing lectures for doctors across the country to educate them about the formula. After a local lecture here in Lafayette, Louisiana, a chiropractor named Dr. Ed Chauvin, approached me and told me about a new technique he was using in his practice. It was called Quantum Neurology®. He was the only doctor in our state at that time utilizing this technique.

I remember thinking, *This is probably one of those hocus-pocus techniques with zero scientific merit.* There are so many of these treatment techniques in my field that I really never bought into—mainly because my scientific brain could not make sense of them; however, something about Quantum Neurology® intrigued me. That particular night Dr. Chauvin changed my life, not because he ordered my product, which he did, but because he shared with me his experience with Quantum Neurology®.

Dr. Chauvin was one of the first Quantum Neurologists trained by Dr. George Gonzalez in Quantum Neurology®. In April of 2007, at fifty-one, he returned home from work as though in a fog and recalls that he doesn't even remember driving home. As soon as he stepped inside the house, he collapsed. At the hospital, he had a CT scan and, lo and behold, Dr. Chauvin had a grade 5 brain aneurism (a grade 6 aneurism can cause immediate death) the size of a baseball. This meant that a blood vessel in his brain had swollen up to the size of a baseball, and it was putting enormous pressure on his brain. In a fortuitous turn of events, Dr. Chauvin's college roommate and chief of neurosurgery at West Virginia University, Dr. Julian Bailes, happened to be in Louisiana at the same time that Dr. Chauvin had the aneurism.

Dr. Bailes was one of the pioneers of a surgical procedure for reducing class-5 aneurisms, and he performed the emergency surgery that ultimately saved Dr. Chauvin's life. The harder part was the recovery. Dr. Bailes informed the family that Dr. Chauvin wouldn't recover for a long time, as he had some major neurological deficits. He told them that Dr. Chauvin wouldn't go back into practice—ever—and that they'd have to fire his staff and sell his equipment.

During early recovery, Dr. Chauvin began repeating Dr. Gonzalez's name, so the family called Dr. Gonzalez, the founder of Quantum Neurology®. Graciously, he flew in and began treatment on Dr. Chauvin. Within eight days, Dr. Chauvin was out of the hospital, and within less than five weeks he was back into practice full time, doing everything he'd done before. Dr. Chauvin believed that because he had already been strengthening his nervous system with Quantum Neurology® pre-aneurism, he was strong enough to survive the ordeal, and he was able to recover so quickly because Dr. Gonzalez immediately rebooted his nervous system. As you'll see, this is the cornerstone of Quantum Neurology®.

I met the story with skepticism, but something intrigued me enough to get Dr. Gonzalez's videos and his GRT LITE™. The initial videos teach doctors how to strengthen the brain's connections to all the musculature in the body with the GRT LITE™, and I started using this in practice, seeing where people's weaknesses were with respect to their brain-muscle connections. Within a six to eight month period in 2008, I was seeing incredible results. Before, a patient would come in, and I'd do my old procedure and hope for the best; with the new techniques, I could take an area of the body and instantly make it strong.

The gold standard for neurological testing is muscle strength. I began to test patient muscle strength before and after the techniques I was learning, and the difference in strength was exponential. But it wasn't until Christmas Eve day, 2008, that I finally realized the enormity of Quantum Neurology®. Again, it took my dad to convince me. Amongst the myriad neurological problems my dad has suffered over the years, one was weakness in his left foot and toes from a major disc herniation from farm work over 30 years ago. The particular nerve bothering him runs down the leg into the muscle and is called the extensor hallucis longus, which pulls your toe upward. Normally, you have a grade 5 in that muscle, which means it's rock-solid strong against resistance. With my dad's, unfortunately, the disc pushed on the nerve so hard that the toe became weak enough he couldn't lift it. He had surgery to reduce the disc's pressure on the nerve, but the nerve function never returned. The neurosurgeon told my dad he had a permanently damaged nerve and would always experience some weakness.

Well, on Christmas Eve day, 2008, we were at my parents' house, and I asked my dad to again be my guinea pig. Skeptically, he agreed. With the techniques I was learning, there is a specific technique to activate the L5 nerve. I did just that. *Immediately* his left foot began to work again. Both of us were dumbfounded.

Before I was even willing to think about meeting with Dr. Gonzalez in Los Angeles, it took many success stories like this one in my own practice. I had to believe this stuff with my own eyes. In fact, by the time I met him, I was doing things that Dr. Gonzalez hadn't even taught, which is to say that the successes I experienced drove me to keep discovering. Quantum Neurology® wasn't something that I just jumped into feet first. Since that Christmas Eve day in 2008, I have helped more people than I had in the previous ten years combined. My dad's life changed. He could ambulate. He looked more alive than he had in five years.

Dr. George Gonzalez is a chiropractic physician in California. In 1997, Dr. Gonzalez's wife, Lori, developed a terrible, supposedly permanent neurological disease called cauda equina syndrome in which the spinal nerve roots become acutely compressed. He tried everything from conventional medicine to chiropractic, and nothing had worked. Like me, Dr. Gonzalez felt as though he was literally forced to find something to help his wife by himself. Little did Dr. Gonzalez know that he would develop the most amazing neurological rehabilitation technique ever created. Over the first few years of his discoveries, Dr. Gonzalez formed the basic techniques now being taught to doctors. It is taught in various modules. You'll recognize that these follow the same connections I talked about in "The Breaker Box Brain" in Chapter 3.

Module I – Brain to Muscles
Module II – Brain to Skin
Module III – Brain to Organs

In order to become a certified Quantum Neurologist, doctors must take two courses in each module. Because Quantum Neurology® is so new, there are only forty-seven Quantum Neurologists in the entire world, but our techniques are gaining traction.

Exploring Quantum Neurology®'s concepts was like a great awakening. I was making startling discoveries! There was a point at which I was calling Dr. Gonzalez on a weekly basis to share all of my new discoveries. Each of my patients had a different story and new set of variables, and I began to understand what makes nerve health infinitely complex. Everyone's nervous system is different. Structurally, the anatomy is the same, but every person walking through my door has a different set of breakers that are off, or a different group of nerves that may or may not be functioning properly based on their personal history—trauma, genetics, fuel, environment, and other factors. All these things determine collaboratively how many of your nerves will be on or off. You must be able to look at each patient and figure out where their problems are with respect to all their nerves and start repairing the worst problem first.

I remember the day in 2009 that Quantum Neurology® was cemented into my belief system. I had a particular patient with whom I had some amazing results, but as I was working with her—I'd been doing Quantum Neurology® for a year and half or more at that point—she had a weakness in her foot I just couldn't figure out. One day I decided to change things up; I did a new combination of tests, and there it was staring me in the face. I figured out what had gone wrong. I was trained as a chiropractor to correct misalignments in the spinal bones, which helped to relieve pressure on spinal nerve roots, and I didn't have to give up that training to practice Quantum Neurology®. In fact, Quantum Neurology® simply takes those principles a step farther than what we're taught as chiropractors. It specifically looks at the entire nervous system and allows us to figure out where it's not working and how to repair it.

Quantum Neurology® is so advanced that you can help the body *immediately* strengthen the nervous system and validate it with that golden standard of neurological testing: muscle strength. This is an amazing thing we're seeing. So many of my patients have trouble trying to explain to people in the community what we're doing, but they're still referring people like crazy. The ones who come in who are initially skeptical—why wouldn't you be?—aren't after one session. I'm working with the body's most complex network and getting results. It's analogous to going to an automobile mechanic thirty years ago. Mechanics didn't have diagnostic computers so that anyone could diagnose your car's problem and produce a handy solution. You had to do your research to make certain you were taking your car to the most thorough mechanic. Quantum Neurologists are like those pre-computer mechanics. We're at the beginning stages of brain and nerve discovery, and only a few of us really get the concepts and intuitions behind the science. This is precisely why I have people coming to see me from all over the country. It will be amazing when we have the technology to create a computerized methodology of looking at the nervous system, but until then we have manual techniques that work for diagnoses and corrections.

The Superhighway

It's important to visualize the whole body as an integrated organism in order to get a true picture of nerve function and brain-to-body connectivity. One more helpful analogy is to think of the brain as a city, the metropolis everyone needs to go into and out of for daily activities. The brain is connected to a massive, straight interstate (your spinal cord) flowing north to south with constant high-speed traffic. Off this massive superhighway are exits and on-ramps on both sides. Once you take an exit onto a smaller road, there are roads (nerves) that go to all surrounding cities, municipalities, and rural areas. Traffic is always flowing into and out of the major city that is your brain. When one area gets slowed, you get a traffic jam. You might be on a rural highway, so the road blocks don't cause as much trouble. But you can also get a jam in the superhighway. A massive jam like spinal stenosis, where a disc or bone has slipped backward, will pinch the spinal cord and cause serious, acute traffic delays. Spinal stenosis can cause more than neck pain—the analogy's equivalent to multi-car pile-ups and over-turned semis. The cars coming from your foot, stomach, or gall bladder to the brain may not be able to get to their destination as quickly or efficiently because of this massive jam.

Let's look at something as simple as bending your finger. Your finger isn't moving by accident. There has to be a nerve that comes from the brain, down through the spinal cord, through your neck, through your shoulder girdle, through your arm, into your hand and fingers to a group of muscles that bend your finger. Your lumbrical muscle is one of the muscles that flexes the finger and is located in the interior part of your palm. For your finger to bend and be strong, you have to have an excellent signal firing from your brain all the way down into that musculature that's bending your finger. If that wire isn't firing well, then the finger is weak. These are just tiny things the brain has to do every day through all of its nerves. In essence, the body is one giant nerve. I will reiterate: the science behind nerve health is understanding how every part of the body is connected, finding the weakness, and immediately strengthening the electrical conduction through that nerve from the brain back out into the area we're trying to help.

If you came in to my office with a weak bicep, I would test your muscle strength in multiple areas to make sure I include all the wires associated with your problem. Your bicep is located in the front portion of your arm and flexes your elbow. If your brain is connected well, it should be nice and strong when we check the neurological strength there (by performing muscle-strength diagnostics). Normal strength equates to cars flowing quickly out through the metropolis in the brain down through the major interstate of the spinal cord, and exiting off the C6 nerve root exit, through the brachium to the bicep. Conversely, if the cars are not flowing—if there's a traffic jam along the way or a slowed flow of traffic between these points—the bicep won't be as strong as it should. In practice, I would be able to push against that arm, and you wouldn't have the proper strength to push back. As a Quantum Neurologist, I can restore the normal flow of traffic to your bicep within a matter of milliseconds.

The Definition of Injury

What you do today, right now, and every day that you're alive is a function of how well your nervous system is working. If you get into a minor car accident and sustain major injuries, that's a direct result of being neurologically compromised *before* you get into that accident. Or what if you're doing something as simple as picking up a pen you dropped on the floor when your back suddenly goes out? This is also a direct result of how well your neurological system was functioning prior to your picking up the pen. Simply, your brain connectivity made you vulnerable, weak, and susceptible to a major injury.

When I have a new patient in the office, and I'm doing an initial history with them, I always ask if they've ever had any accidents or falls, and new patients, almost without fail, say no. Then I'll ask the question a little differently. I'll ask if they've ever had any accidents *without injuries*. They'll always say something like, "Oh sure," and relate stories of fender-benders or bike accidents or falling down stairs.

I want you to think about something. How is it possible that people believe their nervous systems aren't injured by being hit by a two-ton vehicle in a car crash or falling down a flight of stairs? Even if you don't break bones or get whiplash, you've jarred your body enough to warrant a check-up with a Quantum Neurologist. If you don't take care of that injury, it will remain hidden and you'll keep declining.

This applies to all types of injuries. If you bump your head, there's a likelihood you're going to turn off one of your cranial nerves. If you're on vacation at the beach, and you forget your sunglasses, squinting out in the sun all day for several days, you're going to damage cranial nerve VII, your facial nerve, which allows you to raise your eyebrows. Every time you strain your eyes that way again, your connectivity gets weaker. It's possible that one day six months down the road, you'll wake up with Bell's palsy, unable to control one side of your face. How could that happen? Again, it's a direct result of your pre-injury status. If you weren't aware that your cranial nerve VII was initially functioning at, say, 60 percent, versus the 90 percent to 100 percent that protects us from these mishaps, and you close your eyes to go to sleep night after night, you're stressing your nerves just enough for them to lose the connectivity from brain to face.

We must create a much better definition of *injury*. Very simple things like stubbing your toe or bumping your head can create an injury. It's a possibility every time. If you start with low connectivity and bump your head, you could turn off all of your cranial nerves! When I first started working on my dad, all of his cranial nerves were off. Twelve pairs of cranial nerves are responsible for functions of your eyes, ears, nose, tongue, mouth, jaw, scalp, face, and shoulders. For example, he couldn't tolerate any sound, so if the grandkids were screaming, as kids will, he would rush into the bedroom because he couldn't tolerate certain frequencies of sound. This indicated a problem with cranial nerve VIII, the vestibulocochlear nerve, which goes to your ear and gives you the ability to interpret different sound frequencies as well as body balance.

Because the smallest mishaps can injure you, you need your nervous system assessed. If you're not caring for your nervous system, you're setting yourself up for more problems as you get older. It's crucial to get yourself checked out periodically by a Quantum Neurology® practitioner. We're human. We want to take vacations, have adventures, and work hard. We can't live in a glass box, so we just need to be aware of what's going on in our bodies. The nervous system always needs attention. On a daily basis, Quantum Neurology® has a small group of doctors revolutionizing this technique, with more and more doctors coming on board all the time.

The most important thing you should do in your entire life is take care of your nervous system. That's why a lot of people think *I'm just getting older or falling apart* when they feel sore and unwell. This isn't true at all. Aging is not what you think it is. How you feel right now is a reflection of brain connectivity. Period. Listen to your body. Take care of it. Understand that your body needs vigilant care.

The Hidden Diagnosis = Neurological Weaknesses

As I've mentioned before, nerve health varies by individual—your genetics, how you've fueled your body, injuries, posture. All of these things influence how strong your body is neurologically. So many times, a patient comes in and doesn't realize that he or she has a weakness until I expose it.

Quantum Neurologists use a very specific technique that few doctors yet utilize. Let's look at some elite athlete scenarios: ones in which nerve issues can result in very tangible losses. If one finger on a quarterback's hand isn't 100 percent connected to the brain, that finger is weaker than it should be, causing the quarterback's throws to be less accurate than they could be. Maybe he misses the game-winning touchdown throw by several feet because this finger has a hidden neurological weakness. A Quantum Neurologist can fix that.

Maybe it's a pro baseball player, someone who is generally a good hitter but has experienced a six-month hitting slump. If he has a neurological weakness related to cranial nerve VI, which allows the eyes to track laterally, every time he's setting up to look at a pitch, he's in a weakened neurological state. This is a major reason big-time hitters repeatedly fall into "slumps" whereby they go from hitting the ball every game to repeatedly striking out. A baseball player needs the connection from his brain—through the cranial nerve—into eye to be strengthened before he can make the necessary corrections to his hitting.

In the Office: *A Football Player's Story*

Twenty years ago, it seemed impossible that a 6'5" football player weighing 250 pounds would ever break 4.8 seconds in the 40-yard dash, but in 2011 players of this size run a 4.5! However, faster and bigger players are part of the reason why careers end early, and unforeseen injuries are oftentimes coupled with serious neurological injuries. Getting hit by a 250-pound linebacker, who runs a 4.5 second 40-yard dash, is the equivalent of getting hit by an all-terrain vehicle traveling at 18 miles per hour. Football players encounter hundreds and hundreds of these hits.

I recently treated an elite athlete, a college football player, who had torn his anterior cruciate ligament (ACL) the previous season and was gearing up to get back on the field. Prior to seeing me, he had surgery had gone through serious physical therapy to rehabilitate his knee, and he had been cleared by his doctors to play football. Before starting his senior season, he came in to see me, and little did he know that he had a *major hidden diagnosis.* On his first visit, we went through his body and checked the neurological connections from the brain to both legs. All of the brain connections to his legs were rock solid *with the exception of his left leg* (the same leg as the torn ACL). The L3 is a nerve that primarily goes to the Sartorius muscle, which is the muscle that pulls the foot across the body and flexes the hip simultaneously, and this nerve was in a weakened state. The player's right L3 nerve root was perfect, with a strength level of five. (Remember, we measure on a zero to five strength scale.) His left L3 scored a three out of five, meaning that he literally couldn't pull his foot across his body with any amount of resistance. If he had started playing football again in that condition, he'd only survive without another severe injury out of sheer luck.

This athlete was 6'3", 240 pounds; someone of his stature has an ACL almost the diameter of a dime. How is it possible that a ligament of this diameter could be severed? Is it simply because this athlete was exerting too much force? Certainly that's how the injury manifested, but I believed this athlete already had a hidden diagnosis (neurological weakness) *before* his injury. One of his neurological connections to the musculature in his knee was already weak. That's why some people tear their ACLs and others don't.

In the office, we were able to instantly reconnect the L3 nerve connection from brain to body. The athlete went from not being able to pull his foot across his body while flexing his knee, to being rock-solid five minutes after the treatment. When he returned to the football field for his senior college season, he was strong against tearing his ACL again.

Hidden neurological weaknesses happen to everyone. The brain has to have nerve connections to all the parts in the human body, and sometimes we just don't detect the problem before it causes an injury.

In the Office: *A Golfer's Story*

I have a patient who plays golf at an elite level. He can hit the ball well, but he was having trouble with one particular club, the driver. Every time he picked up his driver, his confidence wavered, and his body created a neurological weakness to that club. In my office, I could put the club into the golfer's hands and observe which breakers shut down in his body through the simple reaction that happened in is brain when he held his club. I then strengthened his nervous system in relation to that club. All I did was tell the golfer's brain to fire to the right part of the body. Once I strengthened his body against that weakness, he immediately became stronger and more neurologically capable of dealing with his driver. Without going into the details, this neurological correction enabled him to finish in the top twenty-five in a tournament for the first time in years. The main reason why so many elite, professional golfers go from winning tournaments to not even making the cut often lies in their hidden diagnoses or neurological weaknesses.

How It's Done: *The Natural Plug-In*

As I've said, take all those bodily stressors, mix them up into life's grab bag, and you've got a host of problems. If only the human body had electrical outlets! Were it so, whenever pain or weakness occurred, we could simply re-energize that area by plugging it in and charging it for a few hours.

As Quantum Neurologists, we have discovered why and how to help your body re-energize itself—without power cords or outlets. We know, for instance, how to find the cause of your headaches and how to repair the root of the problem so that your body will heal itself of headaches. A common cause for headaches is a weak trigeminal nerve (cranial nerve V), which supplies power to all the muscles of the jaw and the skin of the head and face. When the trigeminal nerve has a weak connection the brain, headaches commonly occur. As Quantum Neurologists, we have the ability to immediately restore connectivity through this nerve. Thus, we have helped countless people heal themselves of headaches.

We aim to—and succeed daily—figure out the root of pain, fatigue, and a host of other issues. We uncover how to fix them through specific techniques that find weaknesses in the entire nervous system of each patient. Strengthen the nervous system and the body will heal itself. Let's be clear. *As Quantum Neurologists, we don't heal anything; the body does.* I can't say it enough: All we do is strengthen weaknesses in the nervous system, connecting the brain to the body. Better brain connectivity with all body parts makes the whole body stronger and more efficient, which, in turn, allows the body to heal itself more quickly. Because we can't recharge with a power outlet, we use external energy sources to revitalize your body. Currently, we are using infrared light, the entire visible light spectrum, and zero point energy.

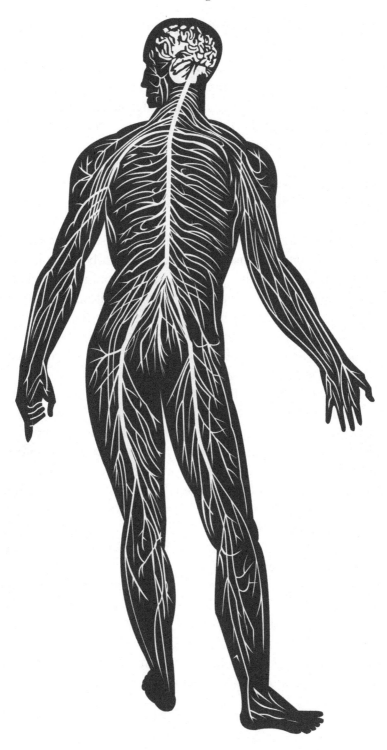

Light and Light Therapy

In Quantum Neurology® we're taught certain techniques in which we use light therapy to strengthen hidden weaknesses in the nervous system. When Dr. Gonzalez began rehabilitating his wife, for instance, he used his invention, the infrared and red GRT LITE ™ to restore her brain's connectivity to all the parts of her pelvis and legs. This ultimately led to his wife living a life without the usually permanent diagnosis of cauda equina syndrome, a life where could foster a pregnancy and deliver a child.

Many doctors use these lights and lasers, but only a few understand *how* to use them, neurologically pinpointing the problem and correcting it. If you have carpal tunnel syndrome, for instance, a doctor can't just put the light on your hand and efficiently correct the problem. With light therapy, we have to first find where a neurological weakness exists. Then we use Quantum Neurology® techniques specific to each nerve in the body and strengthen the weak nerve.

Let's go back to the body. If one of the muscles in the foot is weak, there are very specific anatomical locations we shine the light on to get the nerve to fire back to the foot and make that foot strong again. People are completely dumbfounded the first time we use this light on them, and they instantly get strong. Even when I first started doing this technique, I thought *how is this happening?* But it's really about gaining a deeper understanding of the body.

Your nerves are communicating with your brain through electrical and chemical impulses. The electromagnetic spectrum involves all the different forms of light. The one portion represented in the electromagnetic spectrum that we *can* see is something called the visible spectrum of light, and that consists of the colors we see. There's a whole lot of stuff we can't see in the spectrum, though: microwaves, radio waves, infrared rays, ultraviolet rays, zero point energy.

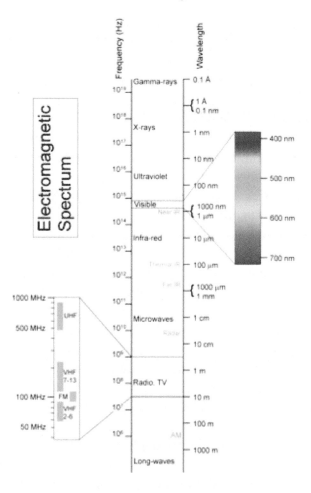

Light is always around us, the center of our being.— It's how our body communicates with itself. In fact, Dr. Gonzalez says in his forthcoming book, *Holographic Healing*, that the human body is actually comprised of two bodies: a LightBody and a Physical Body. He believes the LightBody contains all of our non-physical attributes, including our minds, thoughts, emotions, capacities for love, joy, and spiritual connection. He surmises that the LightBody is the non-physical projected holograph of ourselves, responsible for the connection and communication between ourselves and everything in our universe. In essence, with Quantum Neurology®, we are enhancing the communication between the LightBody and physical body. Better communication between these two bodies means higher neurological function and higher quality of life.

Light is the center of the universe. Without it, there would be no life on earth except bad things like fungus. We are light-emitting creatures. An infrared camera detects infrared light which is normally invisible to the human eye, but it is type of light, nonetheless, that our bodies emit. This is precisely why an infrared light image is seen in the shape of the physical body. Light plays a vital role in everything from religion to quantum physics. In the bible God said, "I am light," plants use photosynthesis to grow, and we use the speed of light to measure seemingly immeasurable movement. Because light is necessary for human existence, we can use it to heal our bodies.

The smallest unit in the electromagnetic spectrum is called a photon. A photon is a unit of light; it's just a tiny particle, but it travels at 670 million miles per hour. That light goes through anything. A great example of this is using a remote control starter for your car. The remote uses an invisible infrared light perfectly capable of traveling through the walls of your house. The light enables you to start your car from inside of your house. Similarly, when light travels through us—if it's the kind of light that our nervous system needs—we are benefitted by the light.

Light therapy is called both phototherapy and heliotherapy, which signify exposure to certain frequencies of light using either artificial or sunlight—any type of light-emitting device. Ancient cultures used sun therapy for healing, but the first person to really start seeing the benefit of light in modern times was a scientist named Dr. Niels Finsen, believed to be the father of light therapy. He used light therapy in a multitude of ways for a dozens of conditions and won the Nobel Prize in Medicine and Physiology in 1903; he specifically won the Prize for treatment of diseases, especially lupus vulgaris, which he used light to help eradicate.

Scientists are just now realizing the power of light and the fact that the human body really does love light. It craves light. Certain types of light help with certain ailments. Quantum Neurology® utilizes the most advanced form of light therapy.

Currently, there are a plethora of light-emitting devices—light-emitting diodes (LEDs), lasers—that are being used in both alternative and traditional healthcare for skin conditions, wound healing, and circadian rhythm therapy; however, as Dr. Gonzalez states:

"Quantum Neurology® targets light in the most effective way; it activates the body's innate healing abilities through the nervous system. Each injury, illness, or condition sets off an alarm within the nervous system. The nervous system activates this alarm to protect the body from further injury. The alarm creates the illusions of pain, decreased range of motion, and dysfunction. Many patients heal with these alarm systems activated. This means that they will experience pain, decreased range of motion, and dysfunction long after their injury, illness, or condition has 'healed.' In many cases this alarm can be active in the patient's body for the rest of his or her life. Quantum Neurology® Rehabilitation turns off the unnecessary alarm systems in the body."

When your brain interprets light in the hypothalamus, in a certain portion of it called the suprachiasmatic nucleus, that gland sends a signal to the pineal gland and makes that pineal gland produce melatonin, which makes you sleep. In other words, when the suprachiasmatic nucleus doesn't see light, it sends the sleep signal. Conversely, when the suprachiasmatic nucleus senses light, it sends a signal for the pineal gland to cease melatonin production, which allows you to stay awake. Our bodies use light; it's no wonder we're able to harness light to reboot our nervous system. Light therapy, when used properly, is the absolute best way to get the nervous system connected.

The light contained in the visible light spectrum includes the colors red, orange, yellow, green, blue, indigo, and violet. We can't see ultraviolet light (UV), microwaves, infrared light, or radio waves. Bees, on the other hand, can see ultraviolet light, and they use this ability to find nectar. Many bird species also have the ability to see ultraviolet light, which they use to help identify the gender of other birds.

When it comes to humans and all the visible frequencies of light, there are no known adverse effects. Think about it: Have you ever heard of someone injuring himself with the light from a powerful flashlight? Conversely, there are plenty of side effects to radio waves and ultraviolet waves. These include everything from cancer to sunburn. Light contained in the visible spectrum is the absolute best form of rejuvenation for our amazing human bodies. This is precisely why we, as Quantum Neurologists, are having so much success by using light to boot up the nervous system.

The Science Behind Zero Point Energy

Another effective nerve-health technology is called Zero Point Energy. Back in the early 1900s, people started talking about atoms, the smallest units in the human body. As I've discussed, if you break the human body down, you'll see that we're a walking mass of trillions of cells, and these cells have to communicate with each other. An even smaller unit of cells is called the atom, so on an even more microscopic level, we're actually walking masses of atoms. If you break it down further, protons, neutrons, and electrons make up atoms. For years, scientists didn't really understand the structure of what was between these protons, neutrons, and electrons. It really wasn't until 1958, when Dutch physicist M. J. Sparnaay started talking about the space in between. At first, this space was considered to be a sort of wasteland, a space with no energy, a vacuum. Sparnaay posited that this space had energy—and he proved it as such. The space in between protons, neutrons, and electrons is actually called zero point energy. This is the basic energy for the human body. With Quantum Neurology®, we have an ability to find the weakness in the nervous system and strengthen it with zero point energy.

In Quantum Neurology®, we use a device that harnesses and emits zero point energy to the area that is deficient in good energy to get your system back up to par. There are people who've spent their whole lives developing instruments that emit zero point energy. Unfortunately—and we've done so much homework on this—there are many companies that sell devices without much therapeutic value. With a good device, however, you can even help yourself at home by wearing a pendant that emits zero point energy the whole time you have it on. A pendant around your neck is located near your lungs and so energizes the air you breathe; it's located near your heart and so energizes your blood; and it also energizes all the food and drink you're putting in your system because it's near your esophagus. These devices have really changed the face of Quantum Neurology® and allowed us to branch into new techniques and get people's systems cranked up faster. {See appendix for my recommendations.}

Zero point energy is such an endless reservoir of energy, and many physicists are starting to recognize its potential. Some are trying to use it to power their houses! We're using it for the human body, but that's just one component of zero point energy. It could possibly be the wave of the future for fueling and energizing our homes, cars, and other devices.

Other Important Techniques

ArthroStim®

In Quantum Neurology®, we also use an instrument called the ArthroStim®. This is an FDA-approved instrument that's been on the market for about twenty-two years, and it's been refined and perfected along the way. It uses a tapping mechanism with very low force to ignite nervous system impulses when they're not firing and also to help restore the flexibility in various joints and reduce subluxations, or slight misalignments, in areas around the spine. This is a much more refined version of the older, more familiar hand manipulation technique that people usually associate with chiropractic care. The ArthroStim® allows us to help restore motion and proprioception to areas of the spine or joints, as well as enhancing the signaling of various nerves to the brain and back. On the spine proper, the ArthroStim® helps to eliminate roadblocks.

Vertical Vibe®

Pure, whole body vibration machines, called Vertical Vibe® machines, use pure vertical vibrations and are absolutely amazing for making the body strong without weights. You can use your body weight on these machines to do more efficient squats than you could on the ground in a hypergravity situation. Your body is thrown into an up-and-down motion that works with gravity and your own weight. Horizontal vibration is hard on your joints, but vertical vibration isn't. We're able to strengthen people quickly using Quantum Neurology® techniques first and then putting their bodies under (good) stress on the machine.

Earth vibrates on its axis. Right now as you read this, you're vibrating at a very low frequency, so the Vertical Vibe® takes that natural vibration and exaggerates it. Believe it or not, bouncing around on bumpy roads in automobiles can trip breakers. So, the Vertical Vibe® actually mimics the kryptonite of driving in a car on a damaged road so that I can observe firsthand whether a patient's breakers are going to trip. Right there in the office, I can strengthen patients against a negative scenario (driving). In addition, standing up normally means that you're contracting only a few muscles, but as soon as you stand on this device, its vertical motion makes more muscles work by contracting continuously. Instead of your brain having to fire to only twenty different muscles on normal ground, when you stand on the Vertical Vibe®, you might have 70–100 muscles that have to contract to keep you stable. You're actually expanding your nervous system, making it more adaptable to various changes it's going to encounter throughout the course of day-to-day life. Vertical Vibe® does the following:

- Increases muscle strength
- Increases growth hormone
- Increases bone density
- Increases athletic skills
- Decreases cortisol levels
- Enhances proprioception (the ability to sense where you are in space)

Brain Time Travel: *More on Mental Stress*

Back to the Future, Planet of the Apes, Bill and Ted's Excellent Adventure, A Christmas Carol, The Time Machine, A Connecticut Yankee in King Arthur's Court, Dr. Who, Austin Powers. I could go on for ages about books and movies that explore time travel. Humans are always imagining time machines or re-imagining the space-time continuum. What we seem to forget is that our brains time travel all day, every day. There are two components to our time travel: conscious and unconscious. If you're vividly and purposefully remembering the time you drove across country with your parents when you were five, that's conscious time travel. You're using your brain to invoke the sights, sounds, and smells of your trip. In the unconscious, time travel is happening that you're not even aware of. Let's say you're at your favorite restaurant and a woman who looks just like your grandmother, who died of cancer when you were twelve, walks in and sits down at the table next to you. You look down at your plate and realize you're eating a meal she liked to cook for you on summer visits. Her death, a traumatic event in your life, triggers your brain to begin a sequence of time travel with images and picture files that have been stored for over a decade.

In the Office:
Dealing with the Death of Parents

I have a patient in her early 40s who was the victim of a huge emotional trauma at a young age. When this patient was in her mid-teenage years, both of her parents died within a two-year span—in their late-40s. This patient proceeded to live her life, get married, and have a successful business. Eventually, though, she began having trouble sleeping. She went to countless doctors, took all kinds of sleep aid medications, but nobody could figure out why she wasn't sleeping, nor was anything helping her sleep. When she came to me, she was desperate to sleep. It took a few sessions, but we deciphered that her conscious mind was healthy:

I would show her pictures of her parents and watch the reaction of her nervous system with her eyes open—her conscious mind's reaction. Then one day, I decided to have her close her eyes and respond to verbal stimuli related to her parents. With her eyes closed, my patient's subconscious mind time traveled to that most painful time in her life and immediately started shutting off neurology that would normally allow her to sleep.

We corrected her connections, strengthened her up, and she immediately started sleeping six to seven hours a night. I can't express how awesome it is to put together the unique neurological puzzle of each patient who comes through my office. Everyone has a different story, different wires, different tripped breakers. We constantly find new Quantum Neurology® methods to further enhance improvement.

Any type of mild to severe emotional trauma is going to be detrimental every time that memory is triggered—unless someone has strengthened your brain. You will become weak to that thought because it was so traumatic to you—and emotional trauma can translate as physical trauma, or nerve disconnection between the brain and body, later in life. The same is true for how your brain deals with future events. Maybe you don't believe in your abilities. Maybe you work for a company and you're doing fine, but you really want to go out on your own. You're petrified and deep down you don't believe you can succeed in running your own business. If you're not confident, that's just another scenario where your brain is weak to that particular thought. If you think a negative thought enough, your brain creates pathways to it: you're time traveling to a negative future.

Let's take a closer look at the brain-foot connection. Say you're in the office for a hidden diagnosis of weak nerves in your foot. I begin by immediately repairing these weak nerves with Quantum Neurology®, and within seconds your foot goes from weak to strong. Then, if I add a stimulus to your brain, say a picture of someone in your past who has died, and the strengthened foot suddenly becomes weak again, that's a prime indication that your brain is particularly weak to that kind of stimulus (an image or memory that stems from the image) as your brain time travels. In other words, every time your brain sees this image, consciously or subconsciously, breakers in your body start to shut off. It's my job to strengthen your brain to those images.

Your brain is going to travel whether you like it or not; it's always thinking. You have to make sure your brain strays strong to *all* possible stimuli. We can't make you forget about bad memories—nor would we want to, as part of being human is negotiating our emotions—so what we have to do is give your brain the girding to deal with this inevitable time travel.

One of the things we've realized is that the human brain is not just thought. It is emotions, feelings, memories, physical connections, electricity, and chemicals flowing in and out of the brain. It's the time travel we do moment to moment. We're not just a body; we're also a mind and a spirit. Our physical bodies and Light Bodies must work in concert in order to maintain optimal health.

Memories and Emotions:
A New Dimension to Quantum Neurology®

I'm a perfectionist. When I have a patient who comes to see me for the first time, and he or she's got, say, twenty different breakers off in the body, I'll turn them back on. If that patient leaves and comes back in two days, and fifteen of those twenty breakers are turned off again, I'll turn them back on. If the same breakers are shut off each time the patient returns, pretty soon I'm going to want to know why. I have seen time and time again that there are always factors in a person's life that create tripped breakers. I don't just want to know *how* to repair patients. I want to know *why*. I want to pinpoint the underlying causes. And even more importantly, I want to know how to keep breakers on.

Every person walking through my door has different breakers tripped in their breaker box. Every person has different types of kryptonite. Mine is different from yours. The stuff that makes you weak is a direct result of your genetics, lifestyle, injuries, history, and past. We have to comb through all of those factors in every individual walking through the door to find answers. The next level of Quantum Neurology® is strengthening patients' neurology to the various forms of kryptonite that affect each individual specifically.

Take the person with the initial twenty breakers switched off. Say we get five breakers to stay on regularly but fifteen breakers are shut off each time she returns to the office. If, as I'm testing this patient's weaknesses, I create a sound frequency with a tuning fork and immediately ten of the fifteen breakers turn off, that's the direct result of a stimulus I've created, but that sound frequency will undoubtedly also exist in her everyday life. I can't stop this patient from hearing a particular sound when she walks out of the office. This is a noisy world we live in. So, I need to make sure I strengthen her to a particular sound frequency so these breakers don't trip.

Another example might be a particular color in the visible spectrum of light. Let's say, every time a particular patient sees the color purple, fifteen breakers turn off. Just like that. These are neurological weaknesses, hidden forms of kryptonite that you'd never know existed. This is the sort of stuff we're uncovering. An excellent example happens in football players, whereby a team gets intimidated and loses badly to another team that they should have easily beaten. Many times this is simply the result of the players' hidden neurological weaknesses to the color of the opposing team's jerseys and/or helmets. In this case, I strengthen the players' hidden weak nerves to the opposing team's jersey and/or helmet color. The results are amazing!

The same goes for calcium pills and bad posture, as we've seen. If a patient comes into the office and tells me that he wants to plant radishes in his garden but can't because of back pain, in the office I will ask this patient to position himself as though he's planting in the garden. I have to see if that position is a form of kryptonite for his particular system. In other words, every time he gets into that position, breakers turn off in his body. Will he go into his garden and trip the same fifteen breakers after our appointments? He will if we don't pinpoint the issue and strengthen the patient to that particular kryptonite.

In the Office: *A Linebacker's Story*

I recently saw another football player, this time a linebacker. His neck was stuck, as if permanently bent forward, in what we call a cervical kyphosis, a term used to describe an abnormal curve in the spine. Every time he bent his neck back, into the normal curvature of the neck, or a lordosis, his breakers would start tripping. As a football player, you'll have your neck jarred backward, especially as a defensive player, where your job is to knock into people. Your neck will be forced into extension. I put him into this tackle position, strengthened up his breakers, and he became more resilient to injury.

As we've discussed, these are pivotal hidden weaknesses and range from elite athletes to someone trying to pull weeds in a garden. So, on an advanced level of Quantum Neurology®, we have to expose these weaknesses in the nervous system and strengthen the body to them.

The most prevalent form of kryptonite I've uncovered so far exists in the emotional category. As we've seen, when you experience a tragedy, like a death in the family, your brain can't let go of the memory of that person. The memory will forever trip your breakers if you don't get your wiring strengthened. Same goes if you want to take a risk and start your own business, but you're too fearful to take the first step. Ultimately, if you could fast forward into the future, you might see that taking the leap would be the best move you ever made, but your brain won't let you because of the fear. Your breakers trip when you experience that fear, keeping you in perpetual stasis.

Take the quarterback who throws an interception and loses the game. Thereafter, every time he time travels and sees that interception, breakers start tripping in his brain. In the office, we would take actual footage from that interception and strengthen his nervous system while he's watching the video, so that if he's ever in that scenario again, about to throw the last pass of the game, the likelihood of him throwing an interception because of tripped breakers is much lower. I feel confident that the teams that win Superbowls and World Series', as well as the individual who wins the Masters and all other major sporting events, are all more neurologically sound, as a whole, than losing teams and individuals.

We are literally beginning to find the root causes of problems and making the brain function as it should. This is the essence of where we're headed with Quantum Neurology®. There are only a handful of doctors who are doing this; once we get more doctors practicing Quantum Neurology®, we'll really tap into the nervous system in ways that nobody has ever imagined.

Conclusion: *Where There's a Will...*

Most of my patients have the *will* to help themselves; they believe in the amazing power of the human body. Unfortunately, I'm also around people who don't have this sort of will. You've heard a lot about my dad in this book, but what I haven't told you is that he is an example of someone who lost the will to help himself, perhaps because he doesn't believe his body is capable of healing itself, or maybe he feels safer with the traditional medicine he grew up using. In the beginning of our neurological rehabilitation sessions, my dad didn't understand what I was doing, but his skepticism was overcome as he saw results—he went from not being able to cognitively function, to being able to spend time with his family, talking and laughing, no longer cringing when the kids ran screaming through the living room. Not to mention, he stayed out of dialysis for almost a four-year period and off of his diabetic medications for almost two years. These facts astounded his team of doctors.

Then, in the beginning of 2011, my dad started eating poorly again; he experienced some serious job stress and house worries. Instead of continuing to take care of himself, he stopped seeing me as frequently. He definitely experienced a shift in will. In 2011, I worked on my dad a total of seven times; in previous years we averaged about twenty visits. Despite multiple heartfelt efforts to persuade him to continue my care, he chose to discontinue care with me. There is a deep sadness in my heart as I have had to sit back and watch his nervous system gradually decline almost back to where it was when I first started working with him.

To my chagrin, my dad is now back on all his diabetic medications and he started dialysis in May of 2011. Once you start this process, your kidneys become dependent on an external filtration system, which makes them lazier than they were in the first place. Without neurological rehabilitation, his health is going backwards; it's a really frustrating process to watch, particularly as a huge chunk of my career has been spent trying to help this man whom I love dearly, and despite all efforts, he has chosen the path to kidney and pancreas transplantation.

I've had to shift gears and realize that I have no control over people's will. I will always give 100 percent, but I can't force 100 percent out of anyone. It's much easier to put your health in someone else's hands. Taking control of your own body requires serious will.

If you want to change your life and foster respect for the amazing human body, you'll see results. Quantum Neurologists are setting a trend in the world right now. We're proving that the body can heal itself of nearly anything and everything. Because you bought this book, I want you to be part of this trend that's going to change history. People just like you will choose health through daily fuel additives, body-and-mind maintenance, and routine repair and strengthening by a trained Quantum Neurologist in your region. You will make better choices in regards to your nervous system. You'll avoid the kryptonite we've talked about. You'll keep all the parts of your body connected to your brain.

This book is a blueprint and should be your primary healthcare manual. You should try every day to strengthen and fuel so that you can avoid synthetic drugs. Find your will to feel good. You're going to feel younger than everyone else around you. Begin the process of neurological rehabilitation that everyone desperately needs.

Appendix

The most difficult part of this process for most people is discipline. It's easy to rush out of the house without taking your morning dose, or to doze off on the couch at night without having done your evening regimen. But let me reiterate that you are in this for the long haul. You are walking around with this amazing machine *that needs the right fuel*....every day of your life! Below are my recommendations for a daily routine and for individual products.

My recommendations for a daily routine:

Take control of your life and give your body the best fuel additives:

DHA: Take three to four softgels in the morning every day (600–800 milligrams per day)

Superfruits GT: Take dosage in the morning before breakfast every day as per my recommended dosage per pound of your body weight:

> 50 pounds = one ounce per day
> 100 pounds = two ounces per day
> 150 pounds = three ounces per day
> 200 pounds = four ounces per day
> 250 pounds = five ounces per day
> 300 pounds = six ounces per day

SeaAloe: Take dosage in the evening after dinner every day as per my recommended dosage per pound of your body weight:

> 50 pounds = one ounce per day
> 100 pounds = two ounces per day
> 150 pounds = three ounces per day
> 200 pounds = four ounces per day

250 pounds = five ounces per day
300 pounds = six ounces per day

Probiotics (PolyFlora for your blood type): Take dosage in the evening, approximately 10–30 minutes after dinner every day as per my recommended dosage per pound of your body weight:

100 pounds or less = one capsule per day
100 – 200 pounds = two capsules per day
200 – 300 pounds = three capsules per day
More than 300 pounds = four capsules per day

Chiropractor's Choice: There are two options:

- Either take three capsules up to three times per day as needed if you experience any aches, pains or soreness.
- Or take two to three capsules two to three times per day every day if you chronically suffer daily with aches, pains, or soreness due to longstanding conditions like arthritis or other inflammatory conditions.

*It is important to remember that Chiropractor's Choice helps support normal low levels of pain, inflammation, and arthritis. It is not intended to cure, prevent or treat anything. Your human body is a machine designed to heal itself.

Pau d'Arco: There are two options:

- Either take one to two milliliters of Pau d'Arco drops on top of tongue immediately after awakening each morning and before bedtime, if you want additional cleansing for your body.
- Or take one milliliter of Pau d'Arco drops on top of tongue immediately after awakening each morning, after each meal, and before bedtime, especially if you chronically suffer from fungal conditions in your nails or skin or recurrent bacterial, viral, or parasitic problems.

When taking SeaAloe and Superfruits GT, it is crucial that you remember the following tips:

- Never drink out of the bottle or cap.
- Always remember to swish Superfruits GT or SeaAloe around in your mouth for a few seconds before swallowing (this will allow absorption to begin immediately).
- Lightly shake the bottle before pouring your dosage.

Furthermore, listen to your body. The moment you start to feel like your body is compromised (e.g., burning nose, fever, aching, congestion), you can easily double or triple this dosage per day until your symptoms decrease.

This will help keep your body's fuel high so you can fight off everything more easily. It is really important to start this mega-dosing the moment you feel compromised in any way.

Daily Fuel Routine for Dr. Chris Cormier (205 pound man):

- Take two milliliters of Pau d'Arco drops on top of tongue immediately after awakening each morning
- Take four DHA softgels with 20+ ounces water (Aquafina)
- Take four ounces of Superfruits GT
- Eat breakfast
- Drink coffee
- Eat lunch
- Eat dinner
- Take four ounces of SeaAloe
- Take two or three PolyFlora capsules
- If I have any soreness or aches or pains, I take Chiropractor's Choice capsules as needed (three capsules taken two to three times daily).
- Take two milliliters of Pau d'Arco drops on top of tongue before getting in the bed each night

Daily Fuel Routine for Dr. Cormier's wife (125 pound woman):

- Take two milliliters of Pau d'Arco drops on top of tongue immediately after awakening each morning
- Take three DHA softgels with 20+ ounces water (Aquafina)
- Take two and a half ounces of Superfruits GT
- Eat breakfast
- Drink coffee
- Eat lunch
- Eat dinner
- Take two and a half ounces of SeaAloe
- Take two PolyFlora capsules
- If she has any soreness, aches, or pains, she takes Chiropractor's Choice capsules as needed (three capsules taken two to three times daily)
- Take two milliliters of Pau d'Arco drops on top of tongue before getting in the bed each night

To order any of my products, please go to my official website, www.TheNerveHealthInstitute.com.

For more details, feel free to contact me or one of my assistants in my office at (337) 456-6555. My office is located in Lafayette, Louisiana. If you need to schedule an appointment to see me, and if you need hotel or flight accommodations, my staff would be happy to assist you. We take great pride in helping as many people as we are capable.

As mentioned in the book, we also offer the *PERSONALIZED Genotype Diet*. After being tested, you'll receive a 30–40 page report with superfoods, neutral foods, and avoid foods suitable only for you as an individual. This is something I have nicknamed the *DNA Based Diet*.

There are a variety of products to suit the needs of all types of individuals. You'll see everything from fuel to posture to exercise as well as educational books and videos:

Weight Loss
Hunger Eliminator Drops
Weight Balancer Drops
DNA Based Diet

Fuel/Nutrition
Probiotics: PolyFlora for your blood type
Chiropractor's Choice
DHA Omega-3 Gelcaps
Pau D' Arco Liquid Drops
Sea Aloe
Superfruits GT

Energy Devices
Zero Point Energy Pendants
Black Tip Zero Point Energy Wands
Grounding Pads

Posture
Therapeutica ® Pillow

Exercise and Fitness
Body Tone 2-Pad Punching Station
Body Tone 4-Pad Kicking Station
Body Tone Heart Rate Monitor
Cardio Pro
Core Inversion Chair
High Density Foam Exercise Blocks
MMA Boxing Tower
Osci Health System
Port-A-Vibe
Pro Inversion Table
Sport Vibe 1000
Sport Vibe 2000
Swiss Chair
Vertical Vibe® Mini Pro 3000
Vertical Vibe® Pro 1000
Vertical Vibe® Pro 2000
Vibra Stack 10000
Vibra Stack 20000
Yogacise

Books

*Holographic Healing – 7 Keys to a Healthy and Energized Life
by Dr. George Gonzalez* (Pre-Order)

*Change Your Genetic Destiny: The Genotype Diet
by Dr. D'Adamo*

Videos

Cranial Nerve X and Zero Point Energy

Lymphatic Therapy with Detox Protocols using the Amega AM Wand

Managing Low Back Pain with Zero Point Energy

Metabolism Weight Loss Strategy with Zero Point Energy– Female and Male

Made in the USA
Las Vegas, NV
01 December 2023

81950283R00089